Essential Oil Recipes Beauty Bible

Over 250 Homemade Organic Skin And Body Care Recipes

(Herbal, Organic and Aromatherapy Essential Oil Recipes For All-Round Natural Body Care)

CADHLA MARIELLE DAVIDS

Limit of Liability

The information in this book is solely for informational purposes, not as a medical instruction to replace the advice of your physician or as a replacement for any treatment prescribed by your physician. The author and publisher do not take responsibility for any possible consequences from any treatment, procedure, exercise, dietary modification, action or application of medication which results from reading or following the information contained in this book.

If you are ill or suspect that you have a medical problem, we strongly encourage you to consult your medical, health, or other competent professional before adopting any of the suggestions in this book or drawing inferences from it.

This book and the author's opinions are solely for informational and educational purposes. The author specifically disclaims all responsibility for any liability, loss, or risk, personal or otherwise which is incurred as a consequence, directly or indirectly, of the use and application of any of the contents of this book.

ISBN-13: 978-1544964614

ISBN-10: 1544964617

DEDICATION

To all who desire to live life to the fullest!

TABLE OF CONTENT

INTRODUCTION 1

ESSENTIAL OIL AND ORGANIC BEAUTY PRODUCTS 5

Figures You Should Know 7

The Essential Oil Art 8

Knowing More About Essential Oils 9

Being Essential-ly Safe 9

Essential Oil In Your Own Beauty Laboratory 10

Essential Oils For Beauty, Hair, Skin and Body Care .. 11

HERBAL, ORGANIC AND ESSENTIAL OIL RECIPES FOR
RELAXATION, MASSAGE AND SPA 13

Lavender Sleep Improvement Oil 13

Body Butter Lotion 14

Lavender Tension Reliever Oil 14

Lavender Mint Relaxation Treat 15

Cedarwood Massage Therapy Oil 16

Epsom Salt Detox Bath With Lavender 17

Child Calming Oil 17

Sauna Therapy 18

Eucalyptus Foot Bath Oil 18

Yoga Meditation Oil 19

Rose Oil Mood Swing & Depression Remedy 21

Mint Cocoa Relaxation Treat 21

HERBAL, ORGANIC AND ESSENTIAL OIL RECIPES FOR DIY
PERFUMES 23

Essential Oils Chart...24

Homemade DIY Perfume With Essential Oils 25

Your Home Perfume Production Factory 28

Jasmine Oil Perfume 30

Tea Tree DIY Deodorant For The Home 31

Lavender Hair Fragrance 31

Lavender Shoe Deodorizer Powder 32

Organic Solid Perfume Recipe 33

Easy Sandalwood Jasmine DIY Perfume....................35

Alpha Male Cologne Recipe.......................................35

HERBAL, ORGANIC AND ESSENTIAL OIL RECIPES FOR THE
FACE 39

Before Bed DIY Makeup Remover Recipe 39

Homemade turmeric skin brightener.......................41

Grapefruit Facial Toner 42

Super All-Natural Anti Wrinkle Cream 43

Apricot Kernel Eye Serum...45

French Green Kaolin Clay Bar 46

Custom-Made Foundation with Sunscreen 47

Rich & Refreshing Face Cleansing Mask...................49

Skin Balancing, Toning and Clarifying Face-wash 50

Lavender Vitamin C Facial Toner 51

Lavender Vitamin C Facial Serum..............................52

Aloe Vera Herbal Infusion Cleanser 53

Silky Face Cream 55

Aloe Dandelion Facial Serum 57

Mint Tea Herbal Face Mist 59

Skin Clearing Face Mask 60

Quick Herbal Steam Treat For The Face 61

Puffy Eye Serum...62

Milky Face-Peeling Mask 63

Wrinkle Removal Cream..64

Anti-Wrinkle Lotion 65

Patchouli Facial Scrub...66

Baking Soda Facial Scrub 67

Beard Care Oil..68

Vitamin C Toning Serum 69

Effective Eye Firming Cream.....................................70

Detoxifying Clay Face Mask 72

HERBAL, ORGANIC AND ESSENTIAL OIL RECIPES FOR THE
MOUTH & LIPS...75

Lemon Infused Lip Balm 75

Lip Healing Balm 76

Cool Breath Mint Oil...............................77

Minty Mouthwash Recipe 78

Teeth Strengthening Toothpaste 79

Whiter Teeth Treat...................................80

Fruity Lip Care Balm 80

Sumptuously Minty Lip Balm 81

Peppermint Lavender Lip Balm................82

Lip Nourishing Lip Balm 83

Minty Rose Syrup Lip Balm 85

Honeyed Lip Scrub & Balm 87

Essential Minty Lip Balm..........................88

Natural Lip Exfoliating Scrub....................89

HERBAL, ORGANIC AND ESSENTIAL OIL RECIPES FOR THE
HANDS AND FEET......................................91

Tired Foot Balm.......................................91

Blistered & Roughened Hand Cream 92

Healing Herbal Hand Salve 93

Revitalizing Herbal Foot Butter................95

Rose Skin Balance Hand Cream 96

Hand Ointment for Men...........................99

Nail Nourishing Oil 101

Winter-proof Cuticle Oil 101

Soothing Foot Oil 102

Calming Cuticle Cream 103

Feet Care Clay Mask..104

Foot Calming Body Butter 106

HERBAL, ORGANIC AND ESSENTIAL OIL RECIPES FOR THE BODY 109

Lavender Herbal Lotion Bars 109

Cellulite Lowering Oil 111

Stretch Mark Healing Oil 111

DIY Skin Toning Oil 112

Pregnant Stomach Balm Bar 113

Plantain Ointment..114

Salt/Sugar Scrub..116

Shea Butter Cream 116

Lavender Shower Gel 119

Cubed Sugar Exfoliating Scrub 120

Body Soothing Lotion 122

Tea Sugar Scrub 125

Skin Nourishing Stretch Mark Cream 126

Talc-Free Body Powder 127

Body Nourishment Lotion 129

Bath Salts Body Treat 130

Lavender Bath Oil..132

All-natural Bath Bombs 133

Body Mollycoddling Wash....................................135

Homemade Skin Splinter Area Ointment...............136

Dry Winter Skin Body Butter 138

Calendula Sun-cream 139

Soothing Diaper Balm..140

Coffee Moisturizing Body Scrub............................142

Tender Skin Shaving Cream 143

Tub Tea Treat...145

Silky Grapefruit Scrub...146

Eucalyptus Shaving Cream...................................147

Concentrated Blemish/Spot Eraser Treatment 148

Natural Homemade Body Salt Scrub......................149

Body Pampering Night Cream 150

HERBAL, ORGANIC AND ESSENTIAL OIL ANTI AGING &
SKIN FIRMING RECIPES..153

Cypress Anti Aging Moisturizing Serum 153

Fresh Honey/Avocado Moisturizer 154

Blood Circulating Salad..155

Daily Anti Aging Toner...156

Agave/Lemon Age Spot Fighter Scrub....................157

Sugar/Almond Anti Aging Face Scrub.....................158

Anti Aging Coconut Deep Conditioner 159

Anti Aging Lip Exfoliator 160

Rice Milk Cleanser..160

Skin Rejuvenating Cream......................................161

Blueberry Granola Anti Aging Exfoliating Mask......163

Age Spots Reduction Oil 164

Anti Aging Skin Scrub 164

Avocado Wheatgrass Anti Aging Mask...................165

Honeyed Anti Aging Scrub.....................................166

Body Anti Aging Oil 167

Eye Anti Aging Roll On...168

Green Tea Anti Aging Cream 169

Daily Anti Aging Eye Cream 171

Homemade Facial Cream 172

Hi-C Face Healing Serum 173

Bentonite Cocoa Mud Mask 175

Rosehip Décolleté Neck & Face Serum 176

HERBAL, ORGANIC AND ESSENTIAL OIL RECIPES TO
FIGHT ACNE, BLEMISHES AND SPOTS 179

ACV Clay Mask 179

Vinegar-Water Anti-Acne Recipe 180

Yogurt-y Spot Removal Mask.................................181

Honey with Cinnamon Face Mask...........................183

Acne Aromatherapy Oil..183

Honeyed tea tree Anti-Acne Face Wash 184

Papaya Anti-Acne Paste...185

Egg whites Scar fading Mask 186

Tea Tree Oil Remedy 187

Orange Peel Paste Mask...188

Banana Peel Face Healing...189

Honey & Strawberries Mix 189

Face Exfoliating Mask...190

Aloe Gel Anti-Acne Remedy......................................191

Lemon Juice Touch...192

Face Clearing Massage Scrub....................................193

Garlic Natural Remedy 194

Steam Face & Beauty Routine Treatment..............194

Sugar Anti-Acne Fighting Scrub................................195

Honeyed Oatmeal Booster 197

Mint Fresh Facial Mask...197

Honey & Avocado Paste 198

Mashed Potato Face Mask 199

Acne Spot & Blemish Treatment...........................200

Face Oil Reducing Tea 201

HERBAL, ORGANIC AND ESSENTIAL OIL SEA SALT
TREATMENT RECIPES 203

Skin Balancing Mask...203

Tender Body Salt Scrub 204

Oil Removing Sea Salt Facial Toner 205

Warm Salt Bath 205

Aloe Gel Salt Scrub 206

Teeth Whitening Powder 207

Anti-Dandruff Salt Treatment................................208

Nail Brightening Salt/Warm Water Solution 208

Salt Soda Mouth Wash 209

HERBAL, ORGANIC AND ESSENTIAL OIL SKIN CLEARING
RECIPES...211

Honeyed Lemon Mix 211

Honeyed Milk Skin Clearing Mix 212

Pine-Turmeric Mix..213

Lemon Soda Skin Clearing Mix................................213

Aloe Gel Moisturizing Skin Clearing Mix.................214

Honeyed Papaya Mix..215

Lemon Cucumber Mix 216

Walnut Skin Clearing Mix 216

HERBAL, ORGANIC AND ESSENTIAL OIL DIY SHAMPOO
HAIR TREATMENT 219

Castile Flavored Shampoo 219

Simple Hair Care Shampoo 220

Baking Soda with ACV Shampoo.............................221

Tea Mint Hair Rousing Shampoo 222

Organic Lavender Shampoo...................................223

Homemade Lavender Rose Shampoo 224

Organic Rose Shampoo 224

Lavender Ylang Ylang Shampoo 225

Aloe Gel Anti-Bacterial Shampoo...........................226

Lavender Hair Care Shampoo 227

Hair Drying Shampoo Mix....................................228

Natural Lemon Shampoo For A Glowing Hair.........229

Hair Anti-Flake Shampoo.....................................230

Lavender Hair Shampoo 231

Queen's Deliciously Scented Shampoo 232

HERBAL, ORGANIC AND ESSENTIAL OIL DIY
CONDITIONER TREATMENT.......................................235

Hair Care Blends; Choosing Carrier Oils Considering
Your Kind Of Hair 236

Herbal Infusion for Simple Herbal Hair Conditioner
....237

Simple Herbal Conditioner 238

Simple Hair Care Oil 240

Homemade Hair Balancing Herbal Rinse................241

Rose Jojoba Hair Conditioner 242

HERBAL, ORGANIC AND ESSENTIAL OIL DIY DEEP
CONDITIONER HAIR TREATMENT 245

Fruity hair conditioner..245

Egg/Mayonnaise Flavored Hair Conditioner...........246

Rosewood Deep Hair Conditioner 247

Mayonnaise/Cinnamon Hair Conditioner 247

Honeyed Mayonnaise Mix.....................................248

Hair Glow Deep Conditioner..................................249

Hot Coconut Hair Mix..251

Light Cream Hair Conditioner 251

Aloe Vera Tea Conditioning Mask..........................252

Castornnaise Deep Conditioner.............................254

Honey Glow Deep Conditioner Hair Treatment 255

HERBAL, ORGANIC AND ESSENTIAL OIL DIY HAIR
DETANGLER 257

Aloe Juice Detangler..257

Natural Aloe Vera leave in & Detangler Mix...........258

HERBAL, ORGANIC AND ESSENTIAL OIL DIY HAIR BUTTER
TREATMENT...261

Rich Shea Hair Butter 261

Hair Butter Moisturizer 262

Complete Hair Butter 263

Tropical Aloe Hair Cream.......................................264

Hair Butter Mask with Pumpkin Seed 265

Cocoa Butter Hair Balm 266

Hair Butter Mask...267

HERBAL, ORGANIC AND ESSENTIAL OIL DIY HAIR OIL
TREATMENT...269

DIY Apricot Hair oil...269

DIY Olive/Coconut Hair Oil Mix..............................270

DIY Castor Hair Oil..270

Hot Coconut Oil Hair Mix......................................271

Egg Oil Hair Mask...272

Hair Growth Oil Inversion......................................273

Hair Oil Mask...274

Carrier Oil Herbal Hair Treat..................................274

Hair Length Oil Mix..275

Hot Oil Treatment for Hair Growth.........................276

Organic DIY Hot Hair Oil Treat...............................277

Beautiful Hair Oil...278

Hair Power Hair Oil..279

HERBAL, ORGANIC AND ESSENTIAL OIL DIY HAIR
GROWTH TREATMENT..281

Mustard Hair Growth Mask....................................281

Essential Blend Growth Oil.....................................282

Hair Force Deep Conditioner..................................283

Rich Herbal Infused Growth Serum..........................284

Hair Health Growth mixture...................................285

Hair Smoothie from the Caribbean..........................287

Apple Cider Vinegar Growth Rinse...........................288

DIY Organic Conditioner (Hair-Growth-Stimulator) 289

DIY Coconut/Honey Cooling Hair Mask...................290

HERBAL, ORGANIC AND ESSENTIAL OIL DIY HAIR GEL
TREATMENT...293

Organic Aloe Hair Gel..293

Aloe Pectin Hair Gel 294

Chamomint Hair Styling Gel....................................295

Matilda's Organic Curls Cream 296

Styling Cream Moisturizer 297

Hair Refreshing Styling Spray..................................298

Glowing Waves Coconut Milk/Oil Conditioner.......299

DIY Leave-In Conditioner..300

Protein Filled Mud mask..301

HERBAL, ORGANIC AND ESSENTIAL OIL DIY NATURAL
SHAVING CREAM 305

Homemade Shaving Cream 305

DIY Shaving Cream 306

HERBAL, ORGANIC AND ESSENTIAL OIL DIY COCONUT
OIL RECIPES FOR HAIR TREATMENT............................309

Coconut Oil Hair Conditioner..................................309

Coconut Oil Scalp Conditioner and Hair Growth
Serum 310

Coconut Oil Anti-Dandruff......................................310

Coconut Oil Frizz Tame..311

Coconut Oil Lice Prevention & Cure Leave-In
Conditioner...312

Coconut Oil Hair Shampoo 313

Coconut Oil Hair Conditioner.................................314

Coconut Oil Dark Hair Color Base 315

Coconut Oil Blonde Hair Color Base.......................316

HERBAL, ORGANIC AND ESSENTIAL OIL DIY HAIR CARE
RECIPES...319

For Oily Hair..319

Scented Hair Aromatherapy Recipe........................320

Dandruff Scalp Treatment 320

Anti-Dandruff Hair Oil 321

INTRODUCTION

There are different essential oils that can fix a headache, inability to sleep, and many other ailments. Needless to say, the use of essential oils is endless! Do you have a Skin and body beauty related problem? There are several essential oils that can fix that.

Essential oils have so many mind blowing advantages for the face, skin, hair and general body care. There are essential oils that work wonder for the skin, they transform, clarify, brighten, moisturize, ad exfoliate the skin. Some are mixed and blended with hair moisturizers, detanglers, conditioners, deep conditioners, oils and gels. The list is endless, below are some beauty essential oils, remedies, treatments and the likes that are used in this book and also added to other natural and organic substances for a healthy beauty routine.

Carrotseed Essential Oil

This oil known to bring the skin back to life, it rejuvenates and helps to smooth the skin. Carrotseed essential oil helps the skin to produce new cells, as a result scars are faded and it makes your skin tone better as your skin becomes older. It has anti-inflammatory, anti-oxidant and anti-wrinkle properties

Geranium Essential Oil

This oil reduces excess skin oil, it has anti-acne properties, enhances your skin's firmness, it is anti-wrinkle, tightens your face and the skin, promotes blood flow wherever you apply this essential oil. Geranium essential oil is known for its healing abilities, healing skin bruise, burns, broken capillaries, cuts, eczema, dermatitis, ringworm and several other skin issues not mentioned here.

Frankincense Essential Oil

This oil works well for all kinds of skin, it has several advantages, it helps the skin fight against bacteria and acne, it has anti-inflammatory properties. It can be used to tone the skin to balance skin tone. It helps regenerate new cells, soothes dry and chapped skin. Fights against and decreases wrinkles on the face.

Myrrh Essential Oil

This oil is wonderful anti-aging essential oil. It enhances the tone of your skin, makes your skin firmer, and reduces wrinkles and lines appearing on your face. It heals damage from the sun, skin rash, eczema and chapped skin.

Lavender Essential Oil

Lavender is a most valuable player when it comes to your organic beauty, skin, hair and body care routine. It works wonders for all types of skins. It has a wonder fragrance, relaxes you and manages the body when stressed. It helps to create new skin cell, works perfectly to renew older skin, and fixes sun scars and spots.

Patchouli Essential Oil

This oil is a great anti-aging essential oil, regenerates new skin cells, reduces wrinkles and lines on your face. It has antibacterial, antifungal and antiseptic properties. It is of great advantage to people with skin problems like dermatitis, eczema, acne and psoriasis.

Neroli Essential Oil

This oil works wonders for older, sensitive and excessively oily skin. It reduces wrinkles and lines across the face. It rejuvenates, grows new cells, prevents and heals stretch marks and exfoliates the skin.

Tea Tree Essential Oil

This oil is known for its great anti-acne, antibacterial, excessive skin oil balancing and healing properties

Rose Essential Oil

This therapeutic oil is known particularly for its help with dry and old skins. It enhances skin texture, balances your skin tone, and heals the skin of various skin conditions like dermatitis and psoriasis.

Ylang Ylang Essential Oil

This oil is one meant for royalty. It smells richly and helps to balance excessive skin oil, grow new skin cells, reduce wrinkles and lines and pampers virtually every type of skin.

ESSENTIAL OIL AND ORGANIC BEAUTY PRODUCTS

Do you know you can make your own beauty products like shampoo, hair conditioner, detangler, body scrubs, body lotions, body butters and so on from the comfort of your own home? Yea maybe not! You probably never thought of it. With the alarming number of store bought cosmetics and beauty products available in the market, it would be difficult to think of anyone taking the time to make DIY beauty and hair products for the personal beauty routine. Well there are numerous advantages to making your own hair care products at home, and I will be explaining some of these advantages below.

a) Its purse friendly; and you cut extra cost.

Just like several other items, homemade hair care products are super cheap compared to store-bought commercial made hair, skin and body care products. Putting numbers into consideration; making your own hair care products is the best option for you, if you have a large family like mine.

b) Your health is wealth.

Several toxic and hazardous chemicals go into the production and packaging of synthetic hair, skin and body care products, even when "natural", "all-natural" is written on the label. Adequate regulations are not put in place to properly regulate, check mate and ensure the safety of most beauty care products we buy and use. Big beauty care and cosmetic producing companies like Suave and Aussie, Pantene among several others use chemicals that are known to cause immunotoxicity, allergies, cancer, and the likes. Needless to say, making your own beauty products and hair care products is the safe way to go, to ensure the safety of the ingredients used and to avoid damage to health on the long term.

c) Efficiency.

So many cosmetics, beauty and hair products make unrealistic promises that never get fulfilled. Making your own beauty and hair products gives you the power and flexibility to create things that would work for you perfectly, your hair type, color and texture.

This is somehow very subjective; but a greater percentage of people say that they have had more results with homemade hair products than store bought commercial brands.

d) Environmental Health.

When you make your own hair care products, you are in charge and your ingredients are natural and organic. Store bought commercial shampoos, conditioner, detanglers and so on contain several tons of harmful chemicals. When natural hair products go down the drain, the environment is safe compared to the synthetic hair products which poisons our water system on the long run.

e) Home Health.

Natural ingredients are safer for your house pipes; they do not damage your pipelines or cause pipeline damage over a period of time. This safety should be put into consideration when considered which hair and beauty products to go for.

Figures You Should Know

1. The average woman will ingest 4 lbs. of lipstick over a lifetime.

2. Only 1155 ingredients out of 10,500 used in beauty, skin and body care products have been publicly evaluated and recorded by the U.S government to be unharmful to the population.

3. The U.S government banned only 10 ingredients that used in cosmetics.

4. The European Union has banned over 1,110 of these ingredients and chemicals.

5. The amount of beauty, skin, personal and body care products said to have at least one cancer causing chemical is placed at 20%

7

6. Only 600 of the several beauty and cosmetics company have signed the compact for safe cosmetics.

7. Cosmetics and beauty products that contains the possible cancer causing impurity 1,4-dioxane are placed at 22%.

8. On a yearly basis, the amount spent on cosmetic surgeries, hair care, skin care, diet products, health clubs and fragrances is placed at $160 billion US dollars.

The Essential Oil Art

The use of essential oils in aromatherapy cannot be overemphasized. Essential oils have the capacity to help our emotions positively. Without using sprays or chemicals, essential oils can fragrance to the home. Some of my greatest high points in the use of essential oils in aromatherapy include nebulizer diffusion, massage, burning oil as incense and heating the oil over a candle.

It is worthy of note to remember that essential oils should always be carefully handled. Essential oils that are not diluted can cause severe skin and health conditions if not handled in the right way; it is therefore important that you are adequately prepared before you begin to use essential oils.

Essential oils should not be applied directly to the skin unless you have diluted the essential oil within carrier oils. Examples of those carrier oils include olive oil, grape seed oil, hazelnut oil or almond oil. Carrier oils help to dilute essential oils so that you can apply to your skin without damaging the oil quality.

Knowing More About Essential Oils

Is it possible to live a natural lifestyle, a world of smelling sweet and out of these world fragrances from natural sources? And also getting to receive the helps of aromatherapy! Yes it is definitely very possible and it is not farfetched; it is possible to have it.

Essential Oils are the oils gotten from plant sources. Examples of essential oils are neroli, peppermint and lemon which can be retrieved in 3 ways:

1. Distillation

2. Cold Press

NOTE: The first two are great ways to extract the oils

3. Solvent Extraction (the use of chemicals to retrieve essential oils)

Being Essential-ly Safe

1. Avoid essential oil contact with your eyes.

2. All essential oils should be stored out of your child's reach.

3. Do not ingest essential oils, especially essential oils like eucalyptus and wintergreen.

NOTE: Some well diluted essential oils can be added to things like toothpaste with caution, but it is widely accepted that essential oils should not be taken internally.

4. There are many essential oils that are toxic to the skin and should be avoided through contact with the skin. Be very cautious. The good news is that most of these toxic essential oils cannot be found in the store.

Essential Oil In Your Own Beauty Laboratory

It is important to test for sensitivity before using an essential oil. It is the best thing to do before you use essential oil for skin care. To test:

Ingredients

1 drop of essential oil

1/2 teaspoon jojoba, olive oil or sweet almond (carrier oils)

Instructions:

1. Combine the essential oil with the carrier oil together

2. Rub the mixture on the inside part of your upper side of your arm and wait a couple of hours.

3. If you are sensitive to the essential oil, an itching or redness will develop.

Essential Oils For Beauty, Hair, Skin and Body Care

The essential oils listed below are some of the very available and least expensive essential oils around.

Lavender: Lavender essential oil works well for hair preparations, used for relaxation, great for all skin types and cleaning products.

Lemon: Lemon essential oil works well in cleaning preparations, lifting moods and sparingly in toners and products for oily skin.

Peppermint: Peppermint essential oil works well for oily/acneic skin remedies, good for lip balms, and cleaning products.

Rosemary: Rosemary essential oil work wells for oily/acneic skin remedies, is good for hair preparations, and cleaning products.

Tea tree: Tea tree essential oil works well for dandruff treatment is great for healing, oily/acneic skin, and cleaning products.

Rose geranium: This essential oil is good for all skin types, making homemade moisturizers and creating perfumes.

Sweet orange: sweet orange essential oil works as very soothing spray for children's room and is good for all skin types.

HERBAL, ORGANIC AND ESSENTIAL OIL RECIPES FOR RELAXATION, MASSAGE AND SPA

Lavender Sleep Improvement Oil

Ingredients

3-4 drops lavender oil

Instructions

1. Get lavender oil,

2. Drizzle 3 to 4 drops of lavender oil on your pillow.

3. It will help eliminate insomnia and help you sleep well.

Body Butter Lotion

Ingredients

Coconut oil

Magnesium oil

Shea butter

Any of your favorite essential oils

Instructions

1. Combine coconut oil, magnesium oil and Shea butter and your favorite oils for moisturizing, together.

2. Mix well.

3. Apply to the body as a moisturizing body lotion.

Lavender Tension Reliever Oil

Ingredients

1 drop lavender oil

Instructions

1. Get lavender essential oil,

2. Add 1 drop of lavender oil to your hands.

3. Rub your hands together, so that essential oil will spread consistently across your palm.

4. Cup your lavender coated hands to your nostrils and allow the scent permeate you and relieve you of anxiety.

Lavender Mint Relaxation Treat

Ingredients

    2-4 drops lavender oil

    2-4 drops chamomile oil

    2-4 drops peppermint oil

Instructions

1. Combine 2 to 4 drops of lavender oil, 2 to 4 drops of chamomile oil and 2 to 4 drops of peppermint oil.

2. Mix well.

3. Apply mixtures to your temple. You will have a cool feel and you will become immediately relaxed on application.

Cedarwood Massage Therapy Oil

Ingredients

3-4 drops lavender or cedarwood essential oil

Unscented oil

Instructions

1. Combine 3 to 4 drops of lavender oil or cedarwood oil with any lotion that is unscented.

2. Mix well.

3. Apply during massage to relax.

Epsom Salt Detox Bath With Lavender

Ingredients

Epsom salt

Lavender oil

Sea salt

Instructions

1. Combine Epsom salts, lavender oil and sea salt together.

2. Mix well.

3. Add mixtures to warm bath.

Your body will be rejuvenated and cleansed.

Child Calming Oil

Ingredients

2-3 drops lavender oil

2-3 drops chamomile oil

Instructions

1. Combine few drops of lavender oil and few drops of chamomile oil together.

2. Mix well.

3. Apply mixture to your child's stuffed animal to sooth and calm them.

Sauna Therapy

Ingredients

2 drops of any of your favorite essential oil

2 cups water

Instructions

1. In a sauna, add 2 drops of any essential oil of your choice into 2 cups of water.

2. Mix to combine well.

Eucalyptus Foot Bath Oil

Ingredients

2-3 drops eucalyptus or lemon essential oil

Water

Instructions

1. Combine 2 to 3 drops eucalyptus oil or lemon oil with warm water.

2. Mix thoroughly.

3. Apply to your feet to soothe.

Yoga Meditation Oil

Ingredients

Sandalwood or lavender essential oil

Citrus oil

Clove oil

Instructions

1. Inhale sandalwood oil or lavender oil before yoga class;

2. Combine citrus oil and clove oil together.

3. Use citrus mixture to clean the yoga mats before meditation. These helps you relax while meditating or during yoga.

Rose Oil Mood Swing & Depression Remedy

Ingredients

Few drops rose oil

Instructions

1. To eliminate mood swings, add rose oil to your inhalations, baths, and diffusers to help boost your mood.

Mint Cocoa Relaxation Treat

Ingredients

1 cup cocoa

2-3 drops peppermint oil

Instructions

1. Make a hot cup of cocoa,

2. Toss in 2 to 3 drops of peppermint oil and mix.

HERBAL, ORGANIC AND ESSENTIAL OIL RECIPES FOR DIY PERFUMES

Aromatic blending is a combination of the depth of science and the creativity of art. A blend could be created primarily for its aroma; therapeutic benefits can still be gotten from such blends, notwithstanding. However, the focus of the blend is not on the therapeutic benefits but on the final aroma that would be gotten.

It is important to adhere to outlined safety precautions during aromatic blending and any other type of blending.

For example, you have to be very careful when handling Bergamot because of its phototoxic properties. You also need to avoid the use of oils that are hazardous, and oils that have contraindications for the conditions you have.

It takes several years to master the science and art of perfumery blending. In aromatherapy blending, only natural ingredients are used compared to perfumery blending and the likes. Ingredients such as, essential oils, CO2s, absolutes, grain alcohol, herbs, carrier oils and water are used. Since aromatherapy blending relies completely on the use of natural and unsynthesized chemicals; aromatherapy blending would not replicate your favorite commercial fragrances perfectly.

Essential Oils Chart

Top Notes

Basil, Anise, Bergamot, Bay Laurel, Citronella, Bergamot
Mint, Galbanum, Eucalyptus, Lavender, Grapefruit,
Lemon, Lavendin, Lime, Lemongrass, Peppermint,
Orange, Spearmint, Petitgrain, Tangerine, Tagetes

Middle Notes

Bois-de-rose, Bay, Carrot Seed, Cajeput, Chamomile
(Roman), Clary Sage, Chamomile (German), Cinnamon,
Cypress, Clove Bud, Elemi, Dill, Fir Needle, Fennel,
Hyssop, Geranium, Juniper Berry, Jasmine, Marjoram,
Linden Blossom, Nutmeg, Neroli, Parsley, Palmarosa, Pine
(Scotch), Black Pepper, Rose Geranium, Rose, Rosewood,
Rosemary, Tea Tree (Common), Spruce, Thyme, {Tea
Tree, NZ (Manuka)}, Yarrow, Tobacco, Ylang Ylang

Base Notes

Angelica Root, Beeswax, Balsam (Peru), Atlas Cedarwood,
Benzoin, Frankincense, Cedarwood (Virginian), Ginger,
Myrrh, Helichrysum (Immortelle), Olibanum, Oakmoss,
Sandalwood, Patchouli, Vetiver, Vanilla

Homemade DIY Perfume With Essential Oils

Making your own perfume isn't as difficult as it sounds. For a long time I wore store bought perfumes, enjoying the beautiful floral scents, having no doubts whatsoever about the perfumes I used.

Not long ago I started to look into the chemicals used in producing my beauty and skin care products. To my shock, I found hidden chemicals in many of beauty and skin care staples which includes my perfume.

While much body sprays, deodorants, antiperspirants and perfumes claims being natural with citrus, floral and exotic fragrances - they are very much synthetic. And more so manufacturers are not obliged to disclose ingredients (such as fragrances and synthetic chemicals), because these ingredients are regarded as production trade secrets.

In some laboratory tests that the Campaign for Safe Cosmetics commissioned, the Environmental Working Group (EWG) discovered

1. Thirty eight secret chemicals in Seventeen name brand fragrances.

These fragrances include;

2. Britney Spears Curious - Seventeen chemicals {not listed},

3. Coco Chanel - Eighteen chemicals {not listed}, and

4. Giorgio Armani Acqua Di Gio - Seventeen chemicals {not listed}.

Many of these name brand fragrances contain secret chemicals that are associated with allergic reactions and endocrine disruption. Secondly most of these chemicals didn't undergo any assessment to check for safety.

This discovery helped me decide to stop buying name brand fragrances and start making my own perfumes.

The Perfume Basics

Making your own perfume is not a herculean task as it may seem. It takes few essential oils and few base ingredients to make that fragrant blend you have always wanted.

The fragrance of a perfume has three classifications. The fragrance is classified into what is called "notes".

There are three notes, such as;

1. The Top Note:

This is the first impression you get from the perfume, it is always light and it evaporates very quickly.

Examples are lemon, grapefruit, orange, lime, citronella, tangerine, bergamot, lavender, eucalyptus, peppermint, lemongrass and spearmint.

2. The Middle Note

This is the major fragrance of the perfume, it is soft, sweet and calm, and it comes out few minutes after the top notes.

Examples are chamomile, clove, cinnamon, cypress, geranium, fennel, jasmine, marjoram, juniper, neroli, pine, nutmeg, fir, rosemary, rose, tea tree, spruce, ylang ylang and thyme.

3. The Base Note

This is the rich part and deep fragrance of the perfume, and most times a musk fragrance.

Examples are cedarwood, ginger, frankincense, helichrysum, patchouli, myrrh, sandalwood, vetiver and vanilla.

Types of Aromas

You can also classify essential oils as aromas or scents

1. Floral: Rose, lavender, geranium, and jasmine

2. Earthy: Patchouli and vetiver

3. Woodsy: Pine and cedar

4. Minty: Peppermint

5. Herbaceous: Basil and rosemary

6. Spicy: Nutmeg, clove and cinnamon.

7. Camphorous: Eucalyptus.

8. Citrus: Lemon and orange.

9. Oriental: Ginger

Your Home Perfume Production Factory

Making your own perfumes is simple based on blending your favorite aromas and mixing with carrier oil. For example floral/spicy or citrus/exotic; below are few blend examples that you can work around.

Grapefruit/Ylang Ylang (Energizing Blend)

1. Combine 7 drops of grapefruit and 4 drops of Ylang Ylang.

2. Mix into a 5ml roller bottle,

3. Add in fractionated coconut oil or sweet almond oil

Fractioned coconut oil is odorless and doesn't become solid when cold.

Lavender/Vetiver/Lemon (Woodsy Blend)

1. Combine 5 drops of lavender, 3 drops of vetiver and 4 drops of lemon.

2. Mix into a 5ml roller bottle,

3. Add in fractionated coconut oil or sweet almond oil

Fractioned coconut oil is odorless and doesn't become solid when cold.

Jasmine/Lime (Floral Blend)

1. Combine 7 drops of Jasmine and 4 drops of lime.

2. Mix into a 5ml roller bottle,

3. Add in fractionated coconut oil or sweet almond oil

Fractioned coconut oil is odorless and doesn't become solid when cold.

Lavender/Copaiba/Lime (Sexy Musk Blend)

1. Combine 5 drops of lavender, 3 drops of copaiba and 4 drops of lime.

2. Mix into a 5ml roller bottle,

3. Add in fractionated coconut oil or sweet almond oil

Fractioned coconut oil is odorless and doesn't become solid when cold.

Jasmine Oil Perfume

Ingredients

1-2 drops jasmine essential oil

Instructions

1. Apply 1 to 2 drops of jasmine oil to your wrist. It acts as a fresh natural fragrance.

2. Clove oil and cypress oil can be used as a substitute for men's cologne.

3. Vanilla and lavender oils are perfect for most women.

Tea Tree DIY Deodorant For The Home

Ingredients

Beeswax

Coconut oil

Tea tree, lavender, clove oil or Cedar wood essential oils

Instructions

1. Mix beeswax and coconut oil together,

2. Mix with your favorite oils like tea tree essential oil and lavender essential oil for women, and clove oil or cedarwood oil for men

Lavender Hair Fragrance
This recipe gives a lovely fragrance to your hair.

Ingredient

1 drop of Lavender/Rosemary/Sandalwood

Instructions

1. Choose any one of the essential oils listed in the ingredient list.

2. Apply 1 drop to the bristles of a hair brush.

3. Use hair brush to brush your hair thoroughly.

Lavender Shoe Deodorizer Powder

Ingredients

    4 tbsps baking soda

    5-6 drops Lavender Essential Oil

    4 tbsps cornstarch (preferably Non-GMO)

Instructions

1. Get a mixing bowl,

2. Combine baking soda and cornstarch together in the bowl.

3. Stir in lavender oil gradually until well incorporated.

4. Pour mixture in a well covered container and store in a cool dry place.

NOTE: You can use powder sifters containers.

5. Apply by sprinkling into shoes several hours before wearing the shoes, evening or overnight is a good time. Before putting shoes on, flip shoes over to get rid of contents of the shoes.

NOTE: Be careful when turning shoes over, to prevent the powder from harming the fragile shoe surfaces. You can add 4 more tbsps of baking soda if cornstarch can't be gotten.

Organic Solid Perfume Recipe

Ingredients

Makes: Approx 1 oz. of solid perfume.

1/8 oz. Floral Wax/Beeswax

7 drops Essential Oil

1/2 oz. Jojoba

Instructions

1. Measure in floral wax or beeswax with jojoba into a double boiler.

2. Melt the wax mixture until completely melted.

3. Remove wax mixture from heat and set aside to cool.

NOTE: Mixture shouldn't be allowed to solidify

4. Toss in your favorite essential oil or essential oil blends.

5. Stir thoroughly to incorporate essential oil into the wax mixture.

6. Pour whole mixture into a suitable container.

NOTE: Do not handle containers while it is hot, allow container to cool completely before handling.

7. Apply as you would a regular perfume.

NOTE: If you added any phototoxic essential oils, do not apply to areas that would be exposed to sunlight directly.

8. Store in a cool, dry place. Recipe should not be used beyond 1 to 2 months.

NOTE: Adhere to all essential oil safety precautions when using any essential oil or blend. Always do a skin patch test for essential oils before usage, make sure the essential oils you are using are gentle to the skin.

Easy Sandalwood Jasmine DIY Perfume

Ingredients

9 drops Sandalwood

1 tbsp Jojoba

3 drops Jasmine/Rose/Neroli (anyone that suits you)

Instructions

1. Get a dark colored container,

2. Blend sandalwood, jojoba and anyone of Jasmine, rose or neroli together. Blend well.

3. Dab to your pulse points as you would a regular perfume.

NOTE: Adhere to all essential oil safety precautions when using any essential oil or blend. Always do a skin patch test for essential oils before usage, make sure the essential oils you are using are gentle to the skin.

Alpha Male Cologne Recipe
This is natural, cool and very manly cologne for a man.

Ingredients

2.5 fluid ounces High Proof Vodka or Perfumer's Alcohol

15 drops Bergamot or Mandarin

1 fluid ounces Distilled Water

15 drops Patchouli

4 ounces glass bottle (with a sprayer top)

5 drops Oakmoss Absolute or 2-3 drops Vetiver

1-2 drops of Neroli (If desired)

3 drops Black Pepper or Ginger

5 drops Bay Laurel

Instructions

1. In a clean and sterilized glass bottle, mix water and alcohol.

2. Add in the essential oils and shake thoroughly.

3. Set aside for several days. Shake bottle vigorously twice a day even while cologne is set aside.

TIP: The setting aside helps the oil to blend well and mellow out before usage for the first time.

NOTE: Adhere to all essential oil safety precautions when using any essential oil or blend. Always do a skin patch test for essential oils before usage, make sure the essential oils you are using are gentle to the skin.

4. Shake well before you and apply as you would a regular cologne.

NOTE: Always shake well before each use to avoid essential oils concentration on your skin.

HERBAL, ORGANIC AND ESSENTIAL OIL RECIPES FOR THE FACE

Before Bed DIY Makeup Remover Recipe

Sleeping in makeup is a nightmare; eventually you get up in the morning feeling so out of sorts and itchy. This recipe is easy and quick to help remove make up naturally with your own homemade make up remover pads.

You just wipe off the makeup and you can go to bed happy

Ingredients

4 oz. glass container with cover

1-2 tbsps witch hazel

1/2 tbsp liquid castile soap

1-2 vitamin E capsules

2 drops tea tree oil

30 cotton pads

2 tbsps water

Instructions

1. In a small bowl, combine the witch hazel, liquid castile soap, vitamin E capsules, and tea tree oil together.

NOTE: Using a sterile-pin, pierce the Vit. E capsules to get out the oil.

2. Place 25 cotton pads into the glass container and toss the bowl's mixture over the pads.

3. Lock the lid in place and shake vigorously.

NOTE: If any of the liquid mixture remains, add more pads until all the liquid mixture becomes absorbed.

4. Turn the pads over and add the 2 tbsps of water and lock the lid back in place.

5. Keep in a cool, dry place.

6. Apply by wiping your face with the makeup remover pads. Avoid the eyes area when wiping.

NOTE: This natural make up remover doesn't need to be washed off or rinsed after use.

TIP: You can put a little amount of warmed coconut oil in your hand and rub gently on your eye region, including your eye lashes using regular cotton pads to wipe away. You don't need to wash off or rinse.

NOTE: You can tweak it a little for your skin type. The Vitamin E oil works perfectly for a skin that is oily, and the tea tree oil will fix incessant skin breakouts. A 4 oz jelly jar would do well for packaging, just find anything that is not too tall and has enough room for your cotton pads.

Homemade turmeric skin brightener

This recipe is an easy homemade skin brightener that doesn't cost so much to make. It will rid your skin of age and sun spots. It also help to prevent diseases like cancer of the skin and it has anti inflammatory properties. It is known to reduce face pigmentation, pimples and acne.

Ingredients

1 tablespoon of hard coconut oil

1 tablespoon organic lemon juice

1/4 teaspoon organic turmeric

1 tablespoon of raw and organic honey

Organic witch hazel

Instructions

1. Combine hard coconut oil, lemon juice, turmeric and raw organic honey together, in a small container.

2. Mix thoroughly to combine.

3. Apply to the face, and leave for 10-15 minutes.

NOTE: Apply cream once in a week.

4. Wash off and rinse your face with warm water.

5. Spray witch hazel on your face, and then moisturize your skin as you would with your normal beauty routine.

Grapefruit Facial Toner

Ingredients

1 oz.fl., High Proof Vodka

8 drops Grapefruit Oil

2 1/2 oz.fl., Witch Hazel Hydrosol

4 drops Cypress Oil

4 ounce bottle

4 drops Tea Tree Oil

Instructions

1. In a clean and sterile glass bottle,

2. Combine vodka, grapefruit oil, witch hazel hydrosol, cypress oil and tea tree oil together.

3. Shake well to combine.

4. Shake thoroughly before use.

NOTE: Shaking thoroughly disperses the essential oils and prevents essential oil concentration.

5. Apply to your face after shaking properly with a cotton ball.

NOTE: Do not use drugstore bought witch hazel has it already contains alcohol.

Super All-Natural Anti Wrinkle Cream
Serves as an anti wrinkle, anti aging cream, also works wonders to remove scars.

Ingredients

3 teaspoons rosehip seed oil

2 teaspoons jojoba oil

3 teaspoons tamanu oil

3/4 teaspoon vegetable based emulsifying wax

3/4 teaspoon beeswax

1/2 teaspoon evening primrose oil

5 teaspoons matcha green tea

1 1/2 teaspoon aloe vera

1 1/2 teaspoon witch hazel

3-5 drops of peppermint essential oil

5-8 drops lavender essential oil

1/2 teaspoon wheatgerm oil

Instructions

1. Combine emulsifying wax, jojoba oil and beeswax together into a bowl.

2. Transfer into a double boiler and melt over medium low heat.

3. Once fully melted, take off from heat.

4. Transfer mixture into a refrigerator to semi-solidify.

5. Whisk wheat germ oil, primrose oil, tamanu oil and rosehip seed oil together in another bowl.

6. Transfer into an electric blender to blend.

7. Meanwhile, combine green tea, aloe vera, witch hazel, peppermint essential and lavender essential oil together in another bowl. Stir to combine well.

8. Pour green tea mixture in to the blender in a slow and steady stream at the highest speed of the blender.

9. Blend until blender mixture emulsifies completely.

10. Store in a jar.

Apricot Kernel Eye Serum

This eye serum moisturizes the area surrounding the eyes

Ingredients

2 tsps jojoba oil

2 tsps avocado oil

2 tsps apricot kernel oil

Instructions

1. Combine ingredients into a dropper bottle.

2. Cover bottle shake well to mix.

3. To apply, drop a tiny drop on your palms and use ring finger to apply to the skin area around the eye.

NOTE: Avoid putting serum to the eyes, eye lids or lashes directly or very near the eyes. It could irritate the eye.

4. Apply once a day at night.

5. Refrigerate.

French Green Kaolin Clay Bar

This clay bar rejuvenates your skin, and amplifies your beauty, skin color and freshness

Ingredients

1/3 cup French green clay

1 tablespoon zinc oxide

1/3 cup kaolin clay

2 tablespoons witch hazel

1/8 teaspoon allantoin, if desired

8 grams melted Shea butter

2 tablespoons aloe vera juice

Silicone mold

Instructions

1. Combine the dry ingredients together in a mixing bowl.

2. Whisk ingredients in the mixing bowl; slowly mix in the liquid ingredients.

3. After mixing well, knead until a sticky and stiff paste consistency is reached.

4. Transfer paste into the mold and smoothen the top. Set aside to 2-3 days to dry completely.

5. Turn mold over and place on a wire rack to dry completely for about a week.

6. Wash your face and wet the soap slightly.

7. Apply the wet side of the soap on your face.

NOTE: If the bar dries out, just wet again.

8. Leave it on your face to dry out for few minutes before you rinse off with a moist towel.

9. Apply argan oil after rinse off.

Custom-Made Foundation with Sunscreen

Ingredients

Jojoba carrier oil

Cocoa butter

Shea butter

Vitamin E

Beeswax

Ground cinnamon

Zinc oxide (uncoated, non-nano, non-micronized)

Cocoa powder

Instructions:

1. Combine shea butter, jojoba, cocoa butter, vitamin E and beeswax in a bowl.

2. Stir to combine well.

3. Transfer and melt in a double boiler over medium low heat; stirring frequently.

4. Take off from heat once mixture has melted completely.

5. Set aside for 5 minutes.

6. Measure in zinc oxide, and cinnamon, mixing to incorporate.

7. Measure in little cocoa powder and stir.

NOTE: Stir in little cocoa powder amounts in successions, stirring each time and comparing with your wrist color.

Stop adding extra cocoa powder when the mixture reaches your desired color consistency.

8. Transfer into a container and set aside to cool.

9. Coat lightly when applying.

Rich & Refreshing Face Cleansing Mask

This face mask refreshes and cleanses and helps smooth your face; leaving your face firm with rich ingredients used in the recipe.

Ingredients

1 tablespoon aloe juice

1/4 teaspoon silk peptides, powder, or amino acids

1 teaspoon green tea extract or matcha powder

5 drops jojoba oil

4–6 teaspoon French green clay

Instructions

1. In a small dish, toss in the aloe juice.

2. Whisk in the silk and green tea into the aloe juice in the dish.

3. Measure in the clay slowly, 1 tsp per time, and whisk until a creamy and thick consistency is reached.

4. Measure in jojoba oil and whisk.

5. To apply, rub a rich amount of the mask on your face.

6. Leave for 20 minutes until mask begins to dry.

7. Wash off and apply argan oil to your face.

Skin Balancing, Toning and Clarifying Face-wash

This recipe helps to tone and clarify the skin. It contains all-natural ingredients that are very gentle and would help to maintain the natural balance of your skin.

Ingredients

1 cup previously boiled or filtered water, (at room temperature)

5 tsps jojoba oil or another facial oil of choice

1/4 cup liquid castile soap

1 tsp tea tree oil

2 tbsps raw honey

10 drops rosemary essential oil

15 drops lavender essential oil

Instructions

1. In a small bowl, measure in water, soap, jojoba oil, raw honey, tea tree oil, lavender essential oil and rosemary essential oil.

NOTE: Add the ingredients in the written order in step 1, don't mix up the arrangements

2. Carefully stir mixture until well combined.

NOTE: The honey and castile soap will make the mixture look cloudy.

3. Transfer mixture into a foaming soap dispenser.

4. Apply facial wash once daily before bed time.

NOTE: Castile soap can be really concentrated. Do not use more than 1-2 pumps at a go. Do not use recipe for more than one month.

5. Shake well before each use.

NOTE: You can slightly adjust ingredients to suit your skin type. For a drier skin use lesser castile soap and more oil or water.

Lavender Vitamin C Facial Toner

Ingredients

1/2 teaspoon natural Vitamin C Powder

8 drops lavender essential oil, if desired.

1/4 cup witch hazel extract

Instructions

1. Mix vitamin C powder, witch hazel extract and the essential oil.

2. Mix well until well combined.

3. Transfer ingredients into a dropper bottle, glass bottle or spray bottle.

4. Shake mixture well to mix.

5. Apply using a cotton pad or cloth after you wash your face daily.

NOTE: Vitamin oxidizes quickly. So recipes should be made in little quantities.

Lavender Vitamin C Facial Serum
Works well for a drier skin.

Ingredients

1/2 teaspoon natural Vitamin C Powder

8 drops lavender essential oil, if desired.

Food grade glycerin

Instructions

1. Mix vitamin C powder, glycerin and the essential oil.

2. Mix well until well combined.

3. Transfer ingredients into a dropper bottle, glass bottle or spray bottle.

4. Shake mixture well to mix.

5. Apply using a cotton pad or cloth after you wash your face daily.

NOTE: Vitamin oxidizes quickly. So recipes should be made in little quantities.

If you have really dry skin or don't want to use witch hazel, you can use food grade glycerin in place of the witch hazel. This will produce a serum instead of a toner. Either one should be made in small batches and often because Vitamin C oxidizes so quickly.

Aloe Vera Herbal Infusion Cleanser

This Aloe cleanser befits only royalty. It leaves your skin beautiful, soft and luxurious.

Ingredients

Makes: 1 (4 ounce) Jar

   1/4 cup/5 tablespoons aloe vera gel

   1 tablespoons castile soap

2 tablespoons sweet almond oil

20-60 drops Essential oils

Instructions

1. Pour aloe vera gel into a bottle; use a funnel.

2. Shake bottle to break aloe vera chunks up.

3. Measure in castile soap, sweet almond oil and essential oils into the bottle.

4. Vigorously shake the bottle until contents mixes well.

NOTE: Bottle content may separate if left for a while. Shake before use.

5. Apply by wetting your face with warm water; pour a small but rich dollop of cream on your clean palms.

6. Rub your palms together and start to apply on your forehead and work your way to your cheeks, nose and to your neck.

7. Close your pores by rinsing your face with cool water, using a muslin cloth.

8. Use an unused towel to pat your face dry.

NOTE: If you have dry skin, use 3 tbsps of sweet almond oil and skip the use of castile soap.

For the essential oils, if you have sensitive skin, use 20 drops. You can use any of these essential oils; they work well for these cleanser; lavender, carrot seed or tea tree essential oils.

Silky Face Cream

This recipe leaves your face beautifully rich and healthy. It has an out of this world smooth consistency and velvety feel that makes your skin soft and alive.

Ingredients

¼ cup organic Olive Oil or Calendula Herbal Oil

¼ cup organic Grapeseed Oil

¼ cup organic Sesame Oil

1/16 cup Beeswax pastilles

1/16 cup organic Coconut Oil

½ cup organic Aloe Vera Gel

1 cup organic Hydrosol of your choice

8-15 drops of any favorite essential oil

¼ teaspoon Vitamin E Oil

Instructions

1. Melt beeswax slowly in a stainless steel saucepan until liquefied.

2. In another stainless steel saucepan over very low heat, mix oils together and warm thoroughly.

3. Mix aloe gel and hydrosol in a small bowl.

4. Warm a double boiler, on low heat.

5. Set aside approx. 10 (2 ounce) glass jars with covers.

6. Transfer half of the warmed oil mixture into the top portion of the double boiler.

7. Measure in a quarter ounce of the melted beeswax into the double broiler.

8. Measure in 6 ounces of aloe gel and hydrosol mixture into a blender, with a quarter tsp of vit.E oil.

9. Measure in your favorite essential oils into the blender.

NOTE: For your essential oils, lavender, orange, rose, sandalwood or chamomile essential oils are great options.

10. Cover the blend and blend to combine, for about a minute.

11. Take out the cover's middle portion in your blender.

12. Set the blender to low and very carefully and slowly transfer the wax and warm oil mixture into the center of the "whirling" waters in the blender.

NOTE: It is very important that you are careful about this process. Patiently pour in a very slow thin stream. At first the cream will look very odd but will gradually reach a thick consistency and will be emulsified. At this point, the blender sound will change.

13. Put the blender off.

14. Use a small spoon or spatula to clean mixtures off the insides of the blender and its blades.

15. Mix cream thoroughly.

16. Put the blender on again and blend finally until a fine mixing consistency is reached.

17. Transfer cream into jars that have been set aside, using the spatula where necessary to get all the cream out.

18. Repeat process for second batch.

19. Store in a freezer for 2-3 hours. Label and Apply as necessary.

Aloe Dandelion Facial Serum

Ingredients

½ cup aloe vera gel

1 tbsp dried dandelion leaves and flowers/5-6 fresh dandelion leaves and flowers

1 tsp vitamin E

Instructions

1. Mix dandelions and aloe gel into a blender or food processor.

2. Blend for 5 to 10 times and set aside for 30-60 minutes to steep.

3. Transfer mixture to a cloth strainer or mesh and strain the dandelions from the aloe vera gel.

NOTE: Make sure there are no dandelions remaining after straining. For best results, strain twice.

4. Measure in a tsp if vit. E oil into the mixture.

5. Store in container that is dark and that has a dropper as cover.

6. You can store in a bathroom drawer. It has a shelf life of 6 to 12 weeks.

7. Apply after using your toner and before using your moisturizer. Smooth 8 to 10 drops of this facial serum over your neck, décolleté and face. Allow to dry before moisturizing.

NOTE: Some certain number of people is sensitive to the latex milk found in dandelion. If you find any reaction like rashes on your skin, discontinue usage and tweak recipes, using only leaves.

Mint Tea Herbal Face Mist

This herbal face mist clears the face and gives your skin the deserved shine

Ingredients

1 drop Tea tree oil

2 bags Peppermint tea bags

Pink Himalayan sea salt

1 drop Lavender essential oil

Instructions

1. Boil a cup of strong peppermint tea in a pot.

2. Stir in sea salt and stir to incorporate.

3. Measure in the tea tree oil into the mixture and stir well.

4. Stir in the lavender essential oil and set aside for a while, to cool.

5. Transfer mixture into a spray glass bottle.

Skin Clearing Face Mask

Ingredients

¼ cup brown rice flour

Yogurt

1 heaping tsp hibiscus powder

Aloe vera gel

Instructions

1. In a mixing bowl, measure in hibiscus powder and rice flour together.

2. Transfer into a jar and cover well.

3. Before each use mix 2 tsps of the dry face mask powder with sufficient amount of aloe gel and yogurt till a paste like consistency is reached.

4. Rub a thick layer on your face and leave to dry for 10 to 15 minutes.

5. Wash your face with warm water after 10 to 15 minutes.

Quick Herbal Steam Treat For The Face

With spring approaching, and the skin damages and the cold and nasal congestions of the winter lingering. You can go the old-school way and give yourself a treat with steam for five minutes.

Ingredients

Few cups of water

Any of your favorite fresh herbs (rosemary, basil or mint)

Instructions

1. Wash your face,

2. Place few cups of water until it almost boils.

3. In a large bowl, pour in hot water, measure in a handful of rosemary, basil or mint.

4. Apply by bending over the bowl of fresh herbs and hot water, covering your head with a clean towel.

5. Do this until the steam dissipates or for five minutes.

NOTE: If you don't have access to rosemary, basil or mint, you can toss in peppermint, chamomile or lavender tea bags.

Puffy Eye Serum

Having puffy eyes or dark circles when enough sleep hasn't been gotten is sometimes hereditary. It happens because oxygenated blood pools under the eyes. Your sleeping position can also be a major contributing factor to this condition. This eye serum corrects this condition.

Ingredients

1/2 cup ground coffee

1 tablespoon Avocado oil

Sweet almond oil

Serum bottle

Instructions

1. In a jar that can be well covered, combine ground coffee and sweet almond oil together.

2. Cover the jar well. Make sure it is airtight.

3. Set aside for a week to infuse oils.

4. Strain the oil from the coffee; using a mesh strainer or cheesecloth.

5. Transfer infused oil to another container or jar.

6. Measure in avocado into the oil content and stir until incorporated.

7. Transfer into a jar and cover.

8. Apply few minutes before bed, using your ring finger to apply on the skin area surrounding your eyes.

Milky Face-Peeling Mask

Ingredients

A small jar

2 tbsps milk

1 packet unflavored gelatin

2 drops eucalyptus essential oil or grapefruit essential oil (or your favorite)

Instructions

1. Measure in a full packet of unflavored gelatin into a small mixing bowl.

2. Measure essential oil into the bowl.

3. Stir in the milk into the mixture in the mixing bowl.

NOTE: The mixture will become clumpy.

4. Place mixture in the microwave for 10 seconds.

NOTE: After you microwave mixture, it should not be clumpy, if it is still clumpy, microwave for 5 seconds more; stirring thoroughly.

5. Apply to your face fast, by slathering a finely thin layer on your face.

NOTE: Avoid your brows and your eyes.

6. Once the mask becomes dry on your face, wash it off and follow with it moisturizer.

Wrinkle Removal Cream

Ingredients

2 teaspoons jojoba oil

3 teaspoons apricot kernel oil

1 teaspoon coconut oil

1 1/2 teaspoon beeswax pastilles

3 teaspoons Rosehip seed oil

6-10 teaspoons rose-water

Instructions

1. Combine jojoba oil, beeswax pastilles, coconut oil, rosehip seed oil and apricot kernel oil together.

2. Transfer into a double boiler to melt over medium low heat for approximately 5 to 8 minutes.

3. Stir to combine and set aside to cool for some minutes.

4. Transfer into an electric blender and blend. Measure rose water slowly and in a steady stream into the electric blender as you blend mixture.

5. Blend until a fluffy cream-like consistency is reached.

6. Refrigerate until you want to use.

NOTE: For a very oily skin, increase the rose water amount to 12-20 teaspoons.

Anti-Wrinkle Lotion

Ingredients

3-5 drops sandalwood, lavender, geranium, and frankincense essential oils

Unscented lotion

Instructions

1. Combine 3 to 5 drops of sandalwood oil, lavender oil, geranium oil and frankincense oil together.

2. Mix with a lotion that is unscented.

3. Rub on face; avoid application to the eyes.

Patchouli Facial Scrub

Ingredients

1/4 cup cornmeal

1/4 yogurt

5 drops patchouli, lavender and grapefruit essential oils

Instructions

1. Combine 1/4 cup cornmeal, 1/4 cup yogurt together,

2. Add mixture to 5 drops of patchouli oil, lavender oil and grapefruit oil.

3. Rub on the face, leave for a while, then rinse off.

Baking Soda Facial Scrub

Ingredients:

   1 tbsp baking soda

   1 drop of pure lavender essential oil

   ½ tbsp honey

   1 drop pure frankincense essential oil

Instructions:

1. Mix honey and baking soda together until it is pasty.

2. Toss in frankincense and lavender oils.

3. Open up your pores by placing a warm towel over your face for a minute thereabout.

4. Apply by massaging your skin with facial scrub to your face gently for 3 to 5 minutes in circular motions.

NOTE: Your face may be slightly red for a while; this is because dead skin has been removed from your face.

5. Wash off and rinse with water that is warm.

NOTE: This facial scrub should be used not more than once or twice weekly. To balance your skin pH, it is important that you splash rose water on your face after steps 1-5.

Beard Care Oil

Ingredients

10-12 tbsps sweet almond oil or jojoba oil or apricot oil

2-3 drops tea tree essential oil

2-3 drops lavender essential oil

2-3 drops cedarwood essential oil

8 ounce dropper bottle

5 drops Vitamin E oil

Instructions

1. Combine sweet almond oil and the essential oils into dropper bottle

2. Measure in vitamin E oil.

3. Shake bottle vigorously to mix

4. Apply as needed.

Vitamin C Toning Serum

This homemade serum clears and tones your skin

Ingredients

1/2 tsp natural real food Vitamin C Powder

2 tbsps vegetable glycerine

1 tsp distilled water

A dark colored container to store

Instructions

1. Combine vitamin C powder and water together to dissolve.

2. Measure in the vegetable glycerine.

3. Set aside in a refrigerator for 4 weeks or more.

4. Apply as a toner after you have cleansed

NOTE: Excess Vitamin C can burn the skin if it is highly concentrated. Adhere strictly to instructions; don't add more than specified amount.

Effective Eye Firming Cream

For a sterling eye treatment, this recipe will help give your eyes that super eye firming treatment needed.

Ingredients

Makes: 4 ounces

1/4 cup green tea

1 tablespoon rosehip seed oil

1/8 teaspoon NeoDefend

1/4 teaspoon vitamin E

1 tablespoon sweet almond oil

1 drop carrot seed essential Oil

1 teaspoon emulsifying wax

3 drops lavender Essential Oil

Instructions

1. Fill 2 medium sized sauce pans half way with water.

2. On medium heat, place 1 glass bowl that has a spout into each sauce pan.

3. Measure in rosehip seed oil, wax, sweet almond oil and vit.E oil into one of the glass bowl inside the sauce pan.

TIP: Meanwhile before step 1, brew one cup of green tea

4. Measure in NeoDefend and the brewed green tea into the second glass bowl in the other sauce pan.

5. Heat the mixtures in the two separate sauce pans until the wax melts completely.

7. Take the temperatures of the two sauce pans with a thermometer.

NOTE: Both have to be at same for the cream to set when combined. Otherwise your cream would not set.

8. When both mixtures in the saucepan reach 130°F, pour the green tea mixture into the rosehip seed oil mixture.

9. Combine cream together, using a hand blender.

10. Mix every ten minutes thereabout for 30-60 minutes, until water doesn't separate at the bottom anymore

11. Measure in essential oils into the mixture once it is fully mixed.

12. This cream works well under make up, use morning and night.

Detoxifying Clay Face Mask

Spray your face lightly with toner as the mask begins to dry to prevent red skin and irritation as the clay mask dries off.

Ingredients

4 capsules activated charcoal

½ cup bentonite clay

1 tbsp finely ground oatmeal

1 tbsp finely ground green tea

1 tbsp finely ground hibiscus

1 tbsp finely ground rosehips

Instructions

1. Mix all the powders in a wooden or glass bowl.

NOTE: This is very important; make you use utensils that are non metal. The Betonite clay has negative charges and it can be deactivated if metal utensils are used.

2. Mix thoroughly until finely mixed.

3. Keep in a cool, dry place and store in a plastic or glass jar.

4. Apply by mixing 1 to 2 tsps of the powdered detoxifying face mask with 2 to 4 tsps of hydrosol or water.

5. Set aside for five minutes before applying to your face.

6. Leave the mask on your face for 15 to 20 minutes.

NOTE: from time to time, spray your face with hydrosol, water or toner whenever your face feels tight, dry or itchy.

7. Use a wash cloth and rinse face off, exfoliating your skin gently in the process.

8. To lock in the moisture and close your pores, apply toner and moisturizer after rinsing.

HERBAL, ORGANIC AND ESSENTIAL OIL RECIPES FOR THE MOUTH & LIPS

Lemon Infused Lip Balm

This lip balm heals cold sores

Ingredients

4 tbsps lemon balm infused oil

1/2 tbsp tamanu oil

1 1/2 tbsp of coconut oil

2 scant tbsps beeswax

1/2 tbsp castor oil

15 drops tea tree oil

1 tbsp mango butter/shea butter

2 drops of clove bud oil (if desired, for pain relief)

25 drops of peppermint essential oil

Instructions

1. In a container that can withstand high heat, mix beeswax, lemon balm infused oil, tamanu oil, coconut oil, castor oil, and shea butter/mango butter together.

2. Mix until thoroughly combined.

3. Fill a saucepan partway with water.

4. Transfer the heatproof container into the saucepan over medium low heat and heat.

5. Heat until the container mixture melts completely.

6. Take away from the heat and measure in the tea tree oil, clove bud oil, and peppermint essential oil

7. Transfer into glass jars.

8. Once lip balm sets, cover and keep away from the sun

9. Apply with cotton swabs and avoid dipping your hand twice at go into the lip balm to avoid contamination.

NOTE: This balm can also be used for patches of dry skin and minor scrapes.

Lip Healing Balm
To heal chapped lips

Ingredients

Beeswax oil

Coconut oil

Lavender oil

Instructions

1. Mix beeswax oil, with coconut oil and lavender oil, together.

2. Mix well.

3. Apply to affected body part for healing.

Cool Breath Mint Oil

Ingredients

1 drop peppermint essential oil

Instructions

1. Add 1 drop of peppermint oil.

2. Apply for cool and fresh breathe.

Minty Mouthwash Recipe

Ingredients

6 oz. fl., Water

4 drops Peppermint/spearmint Essential Oil

1-2 oz.fl., Vodka

3 drops Myrrh

8 ounce bottle

Instructions

1. In a bottle, mix water and vodka together.

2. Add in the essential oils,

3. Cover well, and then shake very well.

NOTE: Essential oils do not mix well in water based solutions. Therefore it is necessary to shake well before each use.

4. Apply as you would any regular mouthwash.

TIP: Vodka helps in killing germs and also helps to keep the essential oils emulsified.

Teeth Strengthening Toothpaste

This makes great remineralizing toothpaste for a great wash.

Ingredients

Baking soda

Sea salt

Coconut oil

Xylitol

Peppermint essential oil

Instructions

1. Mix baking soda, sea salt and coconut oil.

2. Mix with xylitol and peppermint oil.

Whiter Teeth Treat

This treat whitens and clears your teeth

Ingredient

Coconut oil

Fresh strawberries

Lemon oil

Instructions

1. Mix coconut oil, fresh strawberries, and lemon oil together.

2. Apply on your teeth.

3. Rinse your teeth off after 2 minutes.

Fruity Lip Care Balm

Ingredients

3 tablespoons coconut oil, unrefined

1 1/2 tablespoon beeswax pastilles

1 tablespoon mango butter

Vitamin E (if desired)

1/2 tablespoon castor oil (if desired, for a glossy look)

Instructions

1. Combine beeswax and mango butter in a small bowl.

2. Transfer into a double boiler and melt.

3. Once beeswax mixture is melted, toss in the coconut oil into the beeswax mixture and melt.

4. Take off from heat.

5. If using, mix in castor oil, vitamin E, and essential oils, and mix well.

6. Transfer into clean and sterile containers.

7. Set aside to cool before use.

Sumptuously Minty Lip Balm

This lip balm recipe is very sumptuous; it will be difficult to keep from licking your lips every now and then.

Ingredients

3 tablespoon coconut oil, unrefined

1 1/2 tablespoon beeswax pastilles

1 tablespoon cocoa butter

25 drops peppermint essential oil

Vitamin E (if desired)

Instructions

1. Combine beeswax, chocolate chips and cocoa butter in a small bowl.

2. Transfer into a double boiler and melt.

3. Once beeswax mixture is melted, toss in the coconut oil into the beeswax mixture and melt.

4. Take off from heat.

5. If using, mix in vitamin E and peppermint essential oil, and mix well.

6. Transfer into clean and sterile containers.

7. Set aside to cool before use.

Peppermint Lavender Lip Balm

Ingredients

3 tablespoon coconut oil, unrefined

1 1/2 tablespoon beeswax pastilles

1 tablespoon organic unrefined shea butter

25 drops peppermint essential oil and lavender essential oil

Vitamin E (if desired)

Instructions

1. Combine beeswax and unrefined shea butter in a small bowl.

2. Transfer into a double boiler and melt.

3. Once beeswax mixture is melted, toss in the coconut oil into the beeswax mixture and melt.

4. Take off from heat.

5. If using, mix in vitamin E and essential oils, and mix well.

6. Transfer into clean and sterile containers.

7. Set aside to cool before use.

Lip Nourishing Lip Balm

Ingredients

3 tablespoons coconut oil, unrefined

1 tablespoon organic unrefined Shea butter

1 1/2 tablespoons beeswax pastilles

6 drops cinnamon leaf essential oil

10 drops peppermint essential oil

1-2 teaspoons beet root powder/alkanet root powder (if desired, for pink/red lip tint)

4 drops clove bud essential oil

Vitamin E (if desired)

Instructions

1. Combine beeswax and unrefined shea butter in a small bowl.

2. Transfer into a double boiler and melt.

3. Once beeswax mixture is melted, toss in the coconut oil into the beeswax mixture and melt.

4. Take off from heat.

5. If using, mix in alkanet root powder, vitamin E, and essential oils, and mix well.

6. Transfer into clean and sterile containers.

7. Set aside to cool before use.

Minty Rose Syrup Lip Balm

Ingredients

1 tbsp shea butter

1/2 tbsp castor oil

2 1/2 tbsps rose infused oil

Powdered alkanet root (for natural color)

1 tbsp beeswax

15-20 drops of peppermint essential oil

Instructions

For Lip Balm Color

1. In a small bowl, measure in few drops of rose infused oil and then mix in a very little amount of powdered alkanet root.

2. Stir to combine until a dark red thick consistency is reached. Put aside.

Making the Lip Balm

3. In another bowl, toss in beeswax, the oils remaining and shea butter.

4. Transfer shea butter mixture into a double boiler over medium low heat, and melt.

5. Take off the heat and mix in the alkanet/rose infused oil paste a little at a time until you reached the kind of color you desire.

NOTE: To get a pink color, use less of the alkanet paste, for more of red, use more of the paste.

6. Measure in the essential oil.

7. Transfer lip balm into tubes.

Honeyed Lip Scrub & Balm

This lip balm heals chapped lips, serves as a lip scrub and also a balm

Ingredients

1 tbsp shea butter

1 tsp almond oil

1 tsp honey

1 tsp beeswax, grated

1 tsp olive oil

3-4 drops vanilla extract

5 white chocolate chips

Lip balm container

Instructions

1. In a small bowl, mix olive oil and almond oil together.

2. Measure in the vanilla extract and mix together.

3. In a bowl that is microwave safe, melt the beeswax in short burst until almost melting completely.

4. Measure in the chocolate chips and continue to heat until both beeswax and chocolate chips are melted totally.

5. Combine the beeswax mixture with the oils in the bowl.

6. Combine until well incorporated.

7. Pour into a clean and sterile lip balm container and allow it set.

NOTE: You can refrigerate to speed up the rate of solidifying.

TIP: a) Rub a little coconut and a little honey to your lips over night to treat chapped lips.   b) With clean fingers, pierce a capsule of vitamin E and apply to cracks in the mouth.

Essential Minty Lip Balm

Ingredients

  2 tablespoons coconut oil

  2 tablespoons beeswax pastilles

  2 tablespoons Shea butter

  8 drops lavender essential oils

  12 drops peppermint essential oils

  Lip balm containers (tubes or metal tins)

Instructions

1. In a dry, clean and sterile mason jar, mix in beeswax, shea butter and coconut oil together.

2. Partly fill a pot with water and place on low heat.

3. Place mason jar into partly filled pot of water,

4. Melt beeswax mixture, stirring from time to time, for 10 minutes or until beeswax mixture melts completely.

5. Turn off the heat and set jar with water and pot aside to cool.

NOTE: Leave mixture in the water, with the heat turned off, so that beeswax mixture wouldn't solidify too fast.

7. Measure in essential oils to the melted beeswax mixture and stir thoroughly to incorporate.

8. Transfer contents into lip balm containers.

NOTE: If any leftover solidified as you were pouring into containers, reheat following the instructions above and transfer to other lip balm containers.

Natural Lip Exfoliating Scrub

This recipe helps to remove dead skin peels from our lips, also helps to reveal the gentle skin beneath.

Ingredients

1 tbsp of white sugar/brown sugar

1 drop of vanilla (if desired)

1 tbsp of honey (or a little coconut oil/olive oil)

Instructions

1. Combine olive oil or coconut oil or honey with brown sugar together.

2. Mix thoroughly until well combined.

3. Transfer into a clean, dry and sterile container.

4. Apply 1-2 times weekly, vigorously rub the scrub on the lips to remove dead skin peels.

NOTE: Let scrub stay for a minute and rinse off with a washcloth that's damp.

5. Use lip balm after applying this scrub.

NOTE: Don't overuse recipe.

HERBAL, ORGANIC AND ESSENTIAL OIL RECIPES FOR THE HANDS AND FEET

Tired Foot Balm

This recipe is the answer for tired feet after a long day's job in work boots, high heels, or even flips flops. It helps to soothe your heels, cracked and dry feet.

Ingredients

Makes: 1 cup

1/4 cup olive oil infused with chamomile and calendula

1/4 cup cocoa butter

1/4 cup lavender infused coconut oil

25 drops peppermint essential oil

25g beeswax, grated

5 drops vanilla essential oil

10 drops lemongrass essential oil

5 drops lavender essential oil

5 drops tea tree essential oil

Instructions

1. Combine grated beeswax, cocoa butter and oils together into a bowl.

2. Transfer into a double boiler over mid-low heat and melt.

NOTE: Don't leave oils to warm excessively.

3. Once double boiler mixture is melted, measure in essential oils and stir to incorporate.

4. Transfer into another container that can withstand heat.

5. Set aside to cool, for 6 to 8 hours.

6. Apply to feet after bathing or showering at night for the next two weeks.

Blistered & Roughened Hand Cream

This recipe is a specialty for hands that are rough with hard work. We love to ride horses and we hold their reins, we have built one thing or the other, we knead dough and all, cleared bushes, shoveled manure, planted and weeded. So this recipe would be a great gift to your parents to help soften their hands that have been roughened by age.

Ingredients

1/4 cup shea butter

1 tbsp beeswax

1/8 cup sweet almond oil

10 drops cedarwood essential oil

10 drops myrrh essential oil

Instructions

1. In a double boiler, combine sweet almond oil, beeswax and shea butter together.

2. Stir to mix from time to time as it melts

3. Take off from heat and set aside 5 to 10 minutes.

4. Measure in the cedarwood and myrrh essential oil.

5. Transfer mixture into a glass container that us small and set aside for few hours to set.

6. Apply to dry hands as frequently as possible, after a long day's work or working with dirt.

Healing Herbal Hand Salve

This hand salve heals the hands; hands roughened by age, hard work and labor.

Ingredients

3 oz. olive oil

1 tbsp lavender buds

2 oz. coconut oil

2 oz. beeswax pellets (white or yellow)

1 tbsp calendula petals, dried

2 oz. shea butter

Instructions

1. In a glass measuring cup, measure olive oil and coconut oil.

2. Place glass jar in a microwave and heat gently.

3. Measure in the lavender buds and dried calendula petals

4. Turn off the heat and set aside for 30 minutes to an hour and then strain.

NOTE: You should warm again if mixture is too thick to strain.

5. Pour the infused oil into the glass measuring cup and then measure in the beeswax.

6. Put mixture into a microwave and reheat.

7. Take out of the microwave and measure in the shea butter.

NOTE: The shea butter will melt fast, make sure you mix thoroughly.

8. Set aside to cool a little and toss in the lavender essential oil.

9. Transfer into a well covered container. Set aside to cool totally.

TIP: It will last for several months, should be used as frequently as you want.

Revitalizing Herbal Foot Butter

This herbal butter revitalizes and uplifts your body and tired feet when applied

Ingredients

1/2 cup (4 oz.) shea butter

4 1/2 tsps (3/4 oz.) beeswax, grated

2 tbsps (1 oz.) avocado oil

1 1/2 tsps non-GMO vitamin E oil

2 tbsps lanolin

30 drops your favorite essential oils

Instructions

1. Combine shea butter, lanolin, beeswax and avocado oil into a small mixing bowl.

2. Stir to combine until well mixed.

3. Transfer into a pot over low heat; heat until completely melted; stirring from time to time.

4. Take off from heat and measure in the essential oil(s) and vitamin E oil.

5. Stir mixture well to incorporate oils.

6. Transfer into a jar. Set aside to cool until mixture solidifies.

7. Apply by massaging a little amount into any part of your body or feet that needs revitalizing and uplifting.

Rose Skin Balance Hand Cream

This cream evens your skin tone, reduces inflammation, and has a mildly astringent effect on open pores.

Ingredients

Makes: about 100ml

1/3 cup (84ml) Rosewater

1/2 teaspoon (2 grams) Sodium Lactate

1/4 teaspoon (1.8 grams) Honey

1/8 teaspoon (0.5 gram) Liquid Germall Plus

1/4 + 1/8 teaspoon (1.5 grams) Geogard Ultra

NOTE: The last 2 ingredients are preservatives if you want to keep the lotion in the refrigerator for more than seven days, or at room temperature.

1 teaspoon (5grams) Sunflower Oil

1/4 teaspoon (1.3 grams) Rice Bran oil

1/4 teaspoon (1.2 grams) Shea Butter

2.5 teaspoon (3.8 grams) Emulsifying Wax

1/8 teaspoon (0.5 gram) Cocoa Butter

1/16 teaspoon (0.2 gram) Xanthan Gum

10-20 drops of (Rose Geranium essential oil, Rose essential oil, and/or (0.5-1 grams) Ylang Ylang essential oil, if desired

20 drops (1 grams) Vitamin E Oil

Instructions

1. In a large mixing bowl, combine rosewater, sodium lactate, honey, liquid germall plus and geogard ultra together.

2. In another bowl, combine sunflower oil, rice bran oil, shea butter oil, emulsifying wax, cocoa butter, xanthan gum, vitamin E oil and the essential oils together.

3. Transfer both contents into two separate mason jars.

4. In a saucepan with a dishcloth at the bottom. Place mason jars in the dishcloth lined sauce pan.

5. Pour water into the saucepan until the content level of the mason jar has been passed slightly.

NOTE: Do not use a microwave please.

6. Bring water filled saucepan to a simmer, and continue simmering for 20 minutes.

NOTE: Both Mason jar contents must be at 176°F temperature.

7. Take out the mason jars carefully trying not to scald your fingers.

8. Slowly and gently transfer the oil jar mixture into the rosewater jar mixture and keep stirring using a spoon.

9. After the oil jar mixture has been completely emptied, use a mini whisk to whisk the whole mixture together for some minutes until a milk creamy consistency is reached.

10. Set cream aside to cool well.

11. Measure in the essential oils and vitamin E oil into the cream mixture and mix to incorporate.

12. Transfer hand lotion into plastic or glass jar and allow the cream to set.

Hand Ointment for Men

Ingredients

1/2 cup calendula, dried

1 cup sweet almond oil/olive oil/apricot kernel oil/sunflower oil

1/8 cup comfrey, dried

7/10 ounce herbal infused oil

1/2 cup avocado oil (if desired)

7/10 ounce beeswax

7/10 ounce coconut oil

7 drops cedarwood essential oil (if desired)

11 drops bay essential oil (if desired, or any of your favorite essential oil)

4 drops lemon balm essential oil (if desired)

Instructions

To make the infusion

1. In a small jar, mix herbs and oils until the jar is filled to the brim.

2. Cover the jar well.

3. Set aside for 2 weeks or a month to infuse oils.

TIP: On the flip side; use warm water bath for an hour or two hours to infuse the oils.

To make the ointment

1. Use a cheesecloth or coffee filter to strain the oil from the herbs.

2. In a double boil, mix beeswax, coconut oil and infused oil together.

3. Melt the mixture totally and set aside for some minutes.

NOTE: Make sure you don't allow the mixture to solidify. Mix well to combine.

4. Measure in the essential oils.

5. Mix well and pour into the glass container. Cover well.

This recipe will stay up to 6 to 12 months or even more.

6. Apply to cracked, work worn and dried hands.

Nail Nourishing Oil

This recipe nourishes and strengthens the nails

Ingredients

10 drops myrrh, frankincense and lemon oil

2 tbps vitamin E oil

Instructions

1. Combine 10 drops of myrrh oil, frankincense oil and lemon oil together,

2. Mix into 2 tbsps of vitamin E oil,

3. Apply to cuticles.

Winter-proof Cuticle Oil

During winter the weather becomes really tough on the cuticles and the surrounding skin. Brush recipe slightly on the cuticles and it will help to keep the cuticles and the surrounding skin soft and winterproofed.

Ingredients

1/2 fluid oz. cranberry seed oil or any cold pressed carrier/vegetable oil that is rich in EFAs

5-8 drops tea tree or lavender essential oils

Instructions

1. Get a nail polish bottle or a small roller bottle or a small bottle with dropper tip,

2. Measure in carrier oil into the cleaned and sterile bottle.

3. Using a pipette or a dropper, measure in the essential oils into the bottle.

NOTE: sandalwood or patchouli essential oils can be a substitute for tea tree or lavender essential oil

4. Shake vigorously to incorporate essential oil well.

5. Shake before each application.

6. Brush nail polish bottle content onto your cuticles and the skin surrounding and massage it in.

NOTE: You can use as frequently as you desire.

7. Store well and don't use beyond 2 weeks after production.

Soothing Foot Oil
This foot oil helps to heal dry and cracked feet

Ingredients

3 drops lavender oil

2 tbsps coconut oil

Instructions

1. Combine 3 drops of lavender oil to 2 tbsps of coconut oil.

2. Rub on dry cracked feet before you go to bed.

3. After application, put some socks on.

Calming Cuticle Cream

This homemade recipe is good for a quality nail care routine, it's a good way to pamper your fingernails.

Ingredients

  1 tablespoon organic beeswax

  5 drops of lavender essential oil*

  2 tablespoons organic shea butter

  2-4 drops of Vitamin E oil

  5 drops of orange essential oil*

Instructions

1. In a mason jar, mix shea butter and beeswax together.

2. Fill 1/3 of a small saucepan partly with water and bring to boiling.

3. Place mason jar into the saucepan with boiling water.

4. Melt beeswax mixture; remove the jar from the water carefully.

5. Measure in the vitamin E oil and essential oils and stir to incorporate.

6. Pour mixture into a small jar, container or canister.

7. Set aside to cool completely and allow hardening.

NOTE: Recipe can stay up to a year or more and doesn't need to be stored in a freezer.

You can skip essential oils in the ingredients if they are not handy.

8. Apply to the skin surrounding the nails and cuticles every night, before going to bed.

Feet Care Clay Mask

Ingredients

Makes: 1 (8 ounce) jar

8 ounce glycerin liquid

2 mL vitamin E oil

3 mL avocado extract

2.4 mL optiphen ND

1 1/2 mL peppermint essential oil

1 cup Rose Clay

1 cup Kaolin Clay

Instructions

1. Combine kaolin clay and rose clay in a large mixing bowl.

2. Whisk bowl's content and set aside.

3. Mix avocado extract, glycerin liquid, peppermint essential oil, optiphen ND and vitamin E oil into another bowl.

4. Mix well to combine.

5. Stir in the liquid mixture into the clay mixture slowly.

6. Continue to stir until a fine consistency is reached.

NOTE: Eliminate all clumps.

7. Transfer mask into an 8 ounce bail jar.

8. Keep in a dry and cool place.

Foot Calming Body Butter

This body butter cream for the feet, is a soothing and calming cream that reduces discomfort and pain of the feet

Ingredients

1/4 cup coconut oil

2 tablespoons calendula petals, dried

3/4 cup shea butter, unrefined

8 drops lavender essential oil

2 tablespoons marshmallow root, dried (already cut up)

8 drops peppermint essential oil

Instructions

1. Preheat oven to 200°F.

2. Turn heat off. Melt shea butter and coconut oil in an oven safe pan on low heat.

3. Toss herbs in, mix until well combined and then place in the oven.

4. Leave herbs for 4 hours or more to steep.

5. Using cheesecloth or mesh strainer, strain herbs from oil; transfer infused oil into a small bowl that you will be using to whip the cream.

NOTE: Warm herb mixture on the stove incase the mixture hardens while in the oven, before straining.

6. Refrigerate oil for a few hours, until it becomes firm but not solid.

7. Take oil out of the refrigerator, and whip oil for half a minute, using a mixer.

NOTE: Use a spatula to mix any part of oil that is stuck at the bottom of the bowl.

8. Measure in essential oils and whip once more, for a minute.

NOTE: At this point, the whipped cream mixture will turn white peaks will be formed; it will look deliciously attractive and tempting to eat. Do not try to taste.

9. Transfer mixture into a clean jar.

10. Soak your feet for a while before bed time, and then apply this foot cream by rubbing it in very well at least 30 minutes before going to bed.

HERBAL, ORGANIC AND ESSENTIAL OIL RECIPES FOR THE BODY

Lavender Herbal Lotion Bars

Ingredients

3 oz. beeswax

20-40 drops of essential oil (if using, peppermint, orange, rose or lavender are great)

1 1/2 oz. shea butter

1 1/2 oz. cocoa butter

3 oz. calendula or any herbal infused oil

Instructions

1. Melt shea butter, cocoa butter and beeswax in a double boiler or a salve-making saucepan on lowest heat you can get.

NOTE: Stir often to keep from burning shea butter mixture.

2. After melting, add calendula oil or any other herbal infused oils.

NOTE: At this point, mixture may start to thicken slightly.

3. Continue to stir while on low heat until the mixture melts totally.

NOTE: It is important to set heat to low to avoid oils from going rancid from too much heat.

4. After you have melted the mixture completely, measure in the essential oils, if using.

5. Transfer mixture into flat sided tin containers or molds.

NOTE: If your environment happens to be as hot as mine, I suggest you use tin, to allow the lotion bars slip out easily.

6. Set aside to cool, until mixture hardens completely.

7. Pop lotion bars out from the tin or molds and use.

8. Store lotion bars in a cool, dry place.

NOTE: If they are in a very hot place, lotion bars will melt.

TIP: In case you can't get herbal infused oil like calendula, you can make use of

3 oz. Grape seed or jojoba oil (or any other cosmetic oil that is easily absorbed by the skin)

Cellulite Lowering Oil

Ingredients

2 tsps of coconut oil

5 drops of grapefruit oil

Instructions

1. Combine coconut oil with grapefruit oil.

2. Massage oil mixture into dimpled areas.

Stretch Mark Healing Oil

Ingredients

5 drops myrrh oil

5 drops frankincense oil

5 drops grapefruit oil

Coconut oil

Instructions

1. Combine 5 drops of myrrh oil, 5 drops of frankincense oil and 5 drops of grapefruit oil together.

2. Mix mixture with coconut oil.

3. Rub on stretch marks

DIY Skin Toning Oil

Ingredients

2 drops lavender oil

2 drop frankincense oil

2 drops geranium oil

8 oz. water

Instructions

1. Combine 2 drops of lavender oil, 2 drops of frankincense oil, and 2 drops of geranium oil.

2. Mix lavender/geranium essential oil mixture with 8 oz. of water.

3. Apply to the skin.

Pregnant Stomach Balm Bar

This bar will help heal the stretch made on your belly during pregnancy

Ingredients

Makes: approx. 2/3 cup

  2 tbsps beeswax

  5 tbsps cocoa butter

  1/2 tbsp carnauba Wax

  1 tbsp macadamia nut oil

  1 tbsp hemp seed oil

  1 tbsp meadowfoam seed oil

  1 tbsp baobab oil

  1 tbsp pomegranate seed oil

  1 tbsp argan oil

  1/2 tbsp vitamin E oil

Instructions

1. Combine carnauba wax, beeswax, cocoa butter, macadamia nut oil, hemp seed oil, meadowfoam seed oil and baobab oil together into a large mixing bowl.

2. Transfer mixture into a double boiler and melt mixture until fully melted; stirring occasionally.

3. Measure in vitamin E oil, pomegranate seed oil and argan oil into the mixture. Stir to melt and incorporate into the mixture.

4. Take mixture away from heat.

5. Transfer mixture into silicone molds.

6. Set molds aside to cool until the mixture solidifies.

Plantain Ointment

Plantain is known for its great healing characteristics. It is used to treat skin irritations, wounds, cuts and scrapes, bug bites and many other skin problems.

Ingredients

Makes: 1/2 cup of ointment

  1/2 cup Olive oil

  1/2 oz. beeswax

1/3 cup dried plantain

Instructions

1. Measure dried plantain and olive oil together.

2. Transfer into a well covered jar and set aside for 2 weeks to infuse the oil.

TIP: a) For an equally great and quicker oil infusion; Place herbs and oils in a very heavy saucepan over very low heat. b) Warm for 1/2 hour. The downside of this other approach is that the integrity of the herbs is compromised a little because of the heat. c) Turn heat off and set covered saucepan aside. This assures us a certain level of effectiveness.

3. Using a mesh strainer or cheesecloth, strain out all the oil from herbs.

4. In a heavy duty saucepan, measure beeswax and melt over very low heat.

5. Once saucepan content begins to melt, pour in the infused oil. Stirring until incorporated.

6. After melting beeswax totally. Transfer mixture into a clean and sterile jar.

7. Set aside to cool before you cover.

NOTE: This recipe will stay up to year.

Salt/Sugar Scrub

Ingredients

2-3 drops of your favorite essential oils

Almond oil

Instructions

1. Combine 2 to 3 drops of any essential oil and almond oil,

2. Add to sugar or rock salt.

Shea Butter Cream

Recipe works perfectly for your skin. This recipe is light, creamy and soft and contains all the nourishment that Shea butter and the other essential oil added in the ingredient has. The consistency of Whipped Shea Butter is similar to that of whipped cream. It is a bit tricky and time consuming to make, but the results are well worth it.

Ingredients

Makes: approx. four (4 oz.) jars of whipped Shea butter

8 net wt. oz. Shea Butter

1/2 teaspoon Vitamin E Oil (preferably T-50 or T-80)

1 tablespoon Jojoba

1/16 teaspoon Pearlescent Mica Powder for Color (if desired)

1/4 teaspoon Essential Oil

Instructions

1. Get an all-temperature jumbo sized mixing bowl,

NOTE: Mixing bowl should be able to withstand hot/cold temperatures.

Your freezer should be able to accommodate the size of the bowl.

2. Boil water in the lower portion of a double boiler.

3. Lower heat to medium high.

4. In the top portion of the double boiler, toss in Shea butter and leave until its melted, stirring frequently.

5 Adjust the temperature of the stove until the Shea butter is at 175°F, using a candy thermometer. Keep heating for 20 minutes at 175°F.

NOTE: Heating higher than 175°F would damage some Shea butter constituents that are nutritive. Be watchful as you heat the Shea butter, Shea butter is flammable.

6. Quickly and carefully transfer heated Shea butter into the jumbo sized mixing bowl.

7. Toss in vitamin E oil and jojoba very quickly.

8. Using a mixer, whisk Shea butter until well mixed for about 5 to 10 minutes.

9. Remove mixing bowl from the freezer, the Shea butter at this time would still be in a liquid stage, though a film of Shea butter that is solid may have formed.

10. Mix Shea butter for 5 to 10 minutes.

NOTE: Repeat the process of mixing Shea butter and returning to the freezer severally. Keep repeating until a firm and consistent Shea butter is gotten. It should look like frosting or whipped cream. It takes a lot of practice to get this things right. Quick freezing the Shea butter for a short while per interval is very important as this will help enhance, expedite and maintain the whipped cream texture of the whipped butter. It is also very important that you don't over freeze the whipped Shea butter, and don't mix for too long either, to prevent whipped Shea butter from becoming gritty.

11. Toss in the essential oils of your choice, once Shea butter has reached frosting or whipped cream consistency.

NOTE: Adhere to all essential oil safety precautions when using any essential oil or blend.

12. Evenly distribute essential oils into whipped Shea butter by mixing well for several minutes.

13. For color, toss in the pearlescent mica powder and combine thoroughly.

14. Scoop into 4 oz. labeled containers; write the date of production on the label.

15. Store in a cool dry place, ensure clean hands when using and don't use for more than a month.

Lavender Shower Gel

Ingredients

70 drops of lavender (or any favorite essential oils of your choice)

7 oz. fl., Shower Gel Base, unscented

8 ounce bottle

Instructions

1. In a mixing bowl, toss in the shower gel base.

2. Blend in lavender oil or any other essential oil you are using.

3. Combine thoroughly.

4. Pour shower gel mixture into an 8 ounce bottle, using a funnel.

NOTE: Adhere to all essential oil safety precautions when using any essential oil or blend. Always do a skin patch test for essential oils before usage, make sure the essential oils you are using are gentle to the skin.

5. Use as you would a regular shower gel.

Cubed Sugar Exfoliating Scrub

Sugar scrubs that are natural are known to always exfoliate and gently polish the skin, and they are far better compared to the abrasive and more synthetic variations available in the market. Their smells are out of this world and very natural.

Most natural sugar scrubs often separate over time, and this can be a nuisance to work with them; though they have so many great advantages. I have written this recipe to the correct the weaknesses found in most natural sugar cube scrubs. This sugar cube scrubs are easy to work with and are very attractive compared to scrubs that separate over time. They last very long when stored in the right way.

Ingredients

Makes: Thirty 1 inch square exfoliating sugar cubes.

11 net weight ounces Soap Base

2 cups White Sugar

4 oz.fl., Cold Pressed Vegetable Oil (use stable lipids like jojoba oil, watermelon seed Oil or   fractionated coconut oil)

1/4 teaspoon Vitamin E oil

1/4 oz.fl., (1 1/2 teaspoon) Essential Oil

Rectangular soap molds

Surgical gloves (needed while working)

Instructions

1. Melt soap base in a double boiler until it is melted completely.

NOTE: Don't overheat so that you dint ruin the soap lather.

2. In a mixing bowl, pour melted soap base.

3. Quickly toss in the Vitamin E oils and vegetable oils into the bowl and stir to combine.

NOTE: You need to be as quick as possible after instruction 1.

4. Toss sugar in and keep stirring.

TIP: Be fast when stirring and tossing in ingredients, because the mixture has tendencies of firming up pretty fast.

5. Knead soap base mixture with your gloved hands.

6. Measure in the essential oils and combine until the essential oil is well incorporated.

NOTE: If the mixture feels very thin, add more sugar until desired consistency is reached.

7. Scoop mixture into soap molds, making sure there are no air traps.

8. Keep aside to set for one hour.

NOTE: The rate at which mixture firms up is dependent on the quality and types of ingredients used. If the mixture appears too thing, refrigerate for a while.

9. Unmold the scrubs before the mixture sets completely; making it very easy to cut the cubes.

10. Cut into 1 inch cubes and allow to firm up for many hours at room temperature.

11. Don't use on skin areas with wounds, abrasions and cuts or if you have eczema. These scrubs can be used on the body and face, avoid the face.

12 Best used within 1 month and 1 ½ months.

Body Soothing Lotion
No greasy after-feel; soothes dry skin and is well absorbed into the skin.

Ingredients

3 tbsps dried chamomile flowers

Almond, olive or grapeseed oil

3 tbsps dried lavender blossoms

2 tbsp beeswax, grated

1/2 cup water

1/8 tsp borax

Lavender tea

10 drops chamomile or lavender essential oils

Instructions

1. Combine almond oil with 1 tbsp of dried lavender blossoms and dried chamomile flowers into a jar with a good cover.

2. Cover well and set aside for 4 weeks to infuse oils.

NOTE: For best results, keep jar where the sun light can reach.

3. Once oils have been infused, use cheesecloth or mesh strainer to strain the flowers from the oil. Squeezing out every little bit of oil from the flower.

4. Bring water in a pot to boiling. Take off from heat after boiling and add the dried lavender blossoms remaining.

5. Lock the pot's lid in place and allow the flavor of the lavender blossoms to be released completely to make lavender tea.

6. Using cheesecloth or mesh strainer, strain the dried lavender blossoms from the water.

7. Combine beeswax and 1/2 cup of infused oil into a double boiler over medium low heat.

8. Heat until the mixture is completely melted.

9. Transfer strained lavender tea into a small pot and bring to boiling.

10. Measure borax into a bowl that can withstand heat and carefully pour in the lavender tea in; stir until borax dissolves completely.

11. In a blender or food processor, whip beeswax/oil mixture.

12. In a careful, steady and gentle stream, pour the borax/lavender tea mixture into the beeswax/oil mixture and continue to mix until the lotion emulsifies completely.

NOTE: Use a spoon to scrape the sides of the food processor from time to time.

13. Measure in the essential oils into the whipped mixture.

Tea Sugar Scrub

It reduces the appearance of skin cellulites.

Ingredients

1 cup of coconut oil or grapeseed, olive oils

1 ½ cup of brown sugar

2 green tea bags

2 tsps of green tea powder

Instructions

1. Boil tea with distilled water, to make one hot green tea cup.

2. Leave aside to cool.

3. In a large bowl, measure in brown sugar, green tea powder and any of the oils in the ingredients, and mix together.

4. Measure in a little amount of the hot cup of green tea into the mixture per time and stir.

NOTE: Repeat step 4 as many times as possible until scrub mixture looks like wet sand from a beach side or grits.

Skin Nourishing Stretch Mark Cream

Nourishing and moisturizing the skin around the thighs and abdomen during pregnancy can reduce and probably completely eliminate the risks of having stretch marks during pregnancy. When the skin is adequately moisturized helps to maintain skin elasticity and prevent stretch marks when loosing significant amounts of weight.

The beauty of the recipe below is that they can be made without the addition of essential oil, as there are concerns as to whether a pregnant woman can be exposed to essential oils.

Cocoa butter comes with a sweet natural aroma, but you may have to consider the deodorized cocoa butter variant if the cocoa butter natural aroma conflicts with the essential oils choice you made.

Ingredients

- 3 net weight oz. Cocoa Butter

- 4 drops Neroli Essential Oil (if desired)

- 1 oz.fl., Avocado Oil (or any other carrier oil of choice)

- 4 oz. jar with a good cover.

Instructions

1. Melt cocoa butter gently in a double boiler.

2. Toss in avocado oil, stirring continuously.

3. Pour the essential oils mixture you are using carefully into a bowl, set aside to cool for a while.

NOTE: Essential oil evaporates easily when exposed to hot temperatures, so it's important to allow it cool for a while.

4. Add essential oils mixture into cocoa butter mixture and stir.

5. Pour mixture into the jar carefully and set aside to cool.

NOTE: The firmness or softness of your mixture is dependent on the room temperature, if the recipe turns out too soft, use lesser oil. If it turns out to firm, add more oil.

This blend can be used with essential oils famed to be helpful with stretch marks or any essential oil that you like.

It is worthy of note that you use only oils that are beneficial and safe for the skin.

6. Apply to your abdomen and upper thighs 2 times per day.

NOTE: Don't apply around the genital area. Stop using if you discover any sensitivity.

Talc-Free Body Powder
This is an absorbent body powder that is free of talc.

Ingredients

30 drops Lavender Essential Oil or any other essential oil you like

4 oz. Body Powder Sifter Container

4 net weight oz. Arrowroot Powder

Instructions

1. In a large mixing bowl, measure in arrow root powder or non GMO (Genetically Modified Organism) cornstarch.

NOTE: Arrowroot is a little more expensive compared to the cornstarch, but it gives a silkier feel. For a skin that is oily, use 1/2 ounce white kaolin powder to substitute the cornstarch/arrowroot powder.

2. Toss in the essential oil and mix well to incorporate.

3. Transfer into a body powder sifter container.

4. Avoid the mucous membranes, the eyes, genitals, mouth and any other sensitive areas of the body.

Apply as you would a regular body powder.

NOTE: Adhere to all essential oil safety precautions when using any essential oil or blend. Always do a skin patch test for essential oils before usage, make sure the essential oils you are using are gentle to the skin.

Body Nourishment Lotion

Ingredients

8 oz.fl., unscented body or hand lotion

10 drops Patchouli essential oil

5 drops Carrot Seed essential oil

20 drops Sandalwood essential oil

Instructions

1. In a mixing bowl, measure in the unscented hand or body lotion.

2. Measure in patchouli oil, carrot seed oil, and sandal wood oil into the bowl.

3. Mix very well to incorporate essential oils into the lotion.

4. With a funnel, transfer bowl's content into a clean and sterile glass bottle.

5. Apply as you would regular body and hand lotion.

TIP: Sandalwood oil, patchouli oil and carrot seed oil helps dry skin, Sandalwood oil and patchouli oils have a rich and lovely aroma when blended together, the carrot seed oil is great for the skin but has a little harsh scent compared to the other two.

NOTE: Adhere to all essential oil safety precautions when using any essential oil or blend. Always do a skin patch test for essential oils before usage, make sure the essential oils you are using are gentle to the skin.

Bath Salts Body Treat

To fix the issue of essential oils not mixing with water, for this recipe we are going to use a solubilizer to minimize the risk of essential oils separating from water and coming in direct contact with our skin. We will be considering Polysorbate 20 or Solubol

Ingredients

3 cups salt (Epsom salt, Dead Sea Salt, Sea Salt, Himalayan Pink Salt)

1 tbsp Jojoba or any other carrier oil

15 drops favorite essential oil(s)

Solubol or Polysorbate 20 Solubilizer

Instructions

1. Mix the essential oil and carrier oil together,

2. Measure in the solubilizer and mix well.

3. In another mixing bowl, add the salt or salts in.

4. Toss in essential oil mixture carefully into the bowl containing salts.

5. With a fork or a spoon, mix salt mixture thoroughly.

6. Get a salt tube, jar or container that covers well.

7. Transfer salts mixture into container and cover well.

NOTE: Salts stored in containers that do not cover well will lose their savor faster.

8. Set aside for a day, and shake well to incorporate essential oils well into the salt mixture.

9. In a running water bath tub, measure in 1/2 to 1 cup of the salts mixture into the tub, and mix thoroughly, to ensure thorough mixing before you enter the tub.

NOTE: a) Add bath salts just before you enter into the tub, to keep the essential oils from evaporating too soon. Make sure the salts dissolves well before entering into the tub, sitting or standing on large chunks of salts can be very painful.

b) Any of the salts listed in this recipe can be used or a combination of these salts. Salts come in many different grain-sizes. Mixing two salts or several of them can make your salts a very pleasant sight to behold. Large grain sizes of salts are more appealing but they can be a little awkward and painful if you sit or step upon few undissolved pieces, and they take a long while before dissolving in the tub.

c) Adhere to all essential oil safety precautions when using any essential oil or blend. Always do a skin patch test for essential oils before usage, make sure the essential oils you are using are gentle to the skin.

Lavender Bath Oil

Ingredients

2 oz.fl., Jojoba or any other carrier oil

Solubol or Polysorbate 20 Solubilizer

20 drops Lavender Essential Oil

Instructions

I. Combine carrier oil and essential oil together.

2. Measure in the solubilizer and mix well.

3. Transfer mixture into a clean and sterile glass bottle.

NOTE: This recipe may be increased.

4. Measure in approx. (7 to 8ml) 1/4 oz of bath oil into your bath water.

5. Mix very well before hopping into the tub, be sure essential oil have dispersed well in the water to avoid sensitization.

NOTE: Every few minutes wave your hands in the water to keep the bath oil mixture from settling in one spot.

All-natural Bath Bombs

This easy to make recipe is very pleasant and appealing when dropped into the tub. After the first and second time, it becomes second nature to make natural bath bombs. Making bath bombs would save you half of the store bought price and it would also help you to be sure that the ingredients are all natural.

Ingredients

1 cup Baking Soda

1/4 teaspoon Powdered Herbs or 1/8 teaspoon Pearlescent Mica {for color and appeal} (not compulsory)

1/2 cup Citric Acid

1/4 - 1/2 teaspoon Jojoba or any other stable carrier Oil

15 drops Essential Oil

Hydrosol or water

Surgical gloves

Instructions

1. Measure in baking soda, powdered herbs or pearlescent mica and citric acid into a large mixing bowl.

2. Stir thoroughly to free clumps.

3. Stir in the essential oil into the large bowl's content, drop by drop.

NOTE: The mixture might fix a little.

4. Gently add in vegetable or carrier oil as you mix the large bowl's contents with your hand.

5. Carefully measure in the hydrosol to the baking soda mixture using a spray bottle, as you keep blending with your hands.

NOTE: Measure in the water or hydrosol drop by drop, it doesn't take much liquid to dampen mixture to the amount needed to form bath bombs. So be careful not to over flood with liquids or moisten too much.

6. Press mixture into molds (you can use melon ballers, or try out soap, ice or candy molds of varying sizes and shapes).

7. Set molds on wax paper and set aside for 1 day to dry.

8. For a fizzy and aromatic bath, you should drop 1-2 bath bombs into your bath tub.

9. Store bath bombs in an well covered bag or container to retain their fizz.

NOTE: Store your citric acid well in a properly covered container to help retain its "fizzing" power.

10. Can stay up to 6 months if stored properly.

NOTE: If you are using strong essential oils such as geranium, adjust essential oil quantity.

Body Mollycoddling Wash

An extremely luxurious and gentle homemade body wash just for the beauty of your skin

Ingredients

1/2 cup coconut milk canned, unsweetened

3 tsp vitamin E oil

2/3 cup castile soap

2 teaspoons vegetable glycerin, if desired

5 drops lavender essential oil

Instructions

1. Mix full-fat unsweetened coconut milk, vitamin E oil, castile soap, lavender essential oil and vegetable glycerin, if using.

2. Mix mixture together until well combined.

3. Transfer into a bottle or jar.

4. Keep refrigerated.

5. Shake well before application.

6. Pour a little on your washcloth and apply.

NOTE: Recipe doesn't have any preservative, and wouldn't stay more than a week due to the coconut milk contained in the recipe. You can substitute olive oil, almond oil or jojoba oil for the vegetable glycerin in the ingredient. When applying, you should be quick because of the coconut milk contained in the recipe.

Homemade Skin Splinter Area Ointment

This recipe is applied directly to sting and bug bite marks or splinter area on the skin.

Ingredients

1/4 cup calendula-infused oil

2 tsps beeswax pellets

1/4 cup coconut oil

3 tsps betonite clay

3 tsps (approx. 15 capsules) activated charcoal

10 drops tea tree essential oil

10 drops lavender essential oil

Instructions

1. Combine coconut oil and beeswax in a small bowl.

2. Mix well.

3. Transfer mixture into a double boiler and melt over medium low heat.

4. Once mixture has melted, measure in the calendular infused oil, betonite clay, activated charcoal, stirring to incorporate.

5. Remove from heat, and set aside to cool.

6. Measure in the essential oils; stirring to combine.

7. Transfer into a well covered glass jar; and store in a dark, cool and dry place.

8. Apply directly on affected skin area every 12 hours until affected skin is corrected.

Dry Winter Skin Body Butter

Ingredients

5 ounce of raw shea butter

4 tbsps solid coconut oil

2 tbsps avocado oil, almond oil, or grapeseed oil

Grapefruit, lavender, frankincense or ylang ylang essential oils

Instructions

1. Combine coconut oil and shea butter in a small bowl.

2. Mix with a mixer and combine thoroughly.

3. Once mixed; measure in avocado oil slowly and keep mixing until well incorporated.

4. Measure in the essential oil(s)

5. Stir to incorporate.

6. Transfer into a clean jar and refrigerate.

Calendula Sun-cream

Ingredients

4 tbsps organic calendula infused oil

4 tbsps neem oil, organic

4 tbsps Aloe Vera Gel

4 tbsps coconut oil

4 tbsps sesame oil

4 tbsps Cocoa Butter or 10 wafers

4 tbsps Beeswax Pastilles

20 drops organic Lavender essential oil

4 tbsps organic Shea Butter

6 ounce containers

Instructions

1. Combine coconut oil, shea butter, cocoa butter and beeswax together in a small bowl.

2. Transfer into a double boiler and melt at medium low heat.

3. After double boiler content is melted, measure in the aloe gel and the oils.

4. Stir until everything blends well. Take off the heat.

5. Measure in vitamin E oil and the essential oils.

6. Stir until well incorporated.

7. Transfer mixture into the prepared containers and set aside to cool before locking cover in place.

NOTE: Wait for an hour before use or over the night preferably.

8. Apply before going out into the sun.

Soothing Diaper Balm

This diaper balm is cloth diaper safe

Ingredients

1 oz. olive oil

1 oz. coconut oil

2 tsps dried chamomile flowers

1 oz. cocoa butter, chopped

1 oz. shea butter

5 drops Tea Tree essential oil

½ oz. beeswax, chopped

2-3 drops Eucalyptus essential oil

2-3 drops Lavender essential oil

2-3 Grapefruit essential oil

2-3 drops Sweet Orange essential oil

Instructions

1. In a small saucepan over low heat, heat olive oil for approx. 10 minutes.

NOTE: Do not bring olive oil to boiling.

2. Toss in the dried chamomile flowers, cook and keep stirring for 10 additional minutes.

3. Remove saucepan from the heat, and set aside for flavors to be released for 1-2 hours.

4. Using a mesh strainer or cheesecloth, strain the chamomile from the oil.

5. Transfer strained oil into a double boiler and measure in shea butter, coconut oil, beeswax and cocoa butter.

6. Melt shea butter mixture until completely melted.

7. Take off from heat and transfer mixture into a bowl.

8. Set mixture aside till it cools.

9. Measure in tea tree, eucalyptus, lavender, grapefruit and sweet orange essential oils. Stir to combine well.

10. Mix mixture on high with a stick blender or stand mixer until the mixture changes from a clear liquid to a whitish solid form.

NOTE: IF in time, this change doesn't occur, or mixture is too watery; refrigerate mixture for 5 to 10 minutes.

11. Scrape bowl sides with a spoon and repeat mixing process.

NOTE: If repeating process doesn't work, measure in more cocoa butter or beeswax until desired thickness is attained.

12. Transfer by scooping into a jar and cover well.

13. Keep in cool, dry place. Do not use for more than 1 year.

Coffee Moisturizing Body Scrub
This recipe keeps your skin soft, hydrated and moisturized.

Ingredients

Makes: 4-5 (4 ounce) Jelly jars

  1 cup coconut oil

  1/3 cup fresh coffee grounds

½ cup sugar

4-5 (4 ounce) jelly jars

2-3 tablespoons olive oil

Instructions

1. Toss in sugar, coconut oil, olive oil and coffee grounds into a medium fairly large bowl.

2. Stir to combine and mix well until thoroughly combined.

3. Transfer mixture into clean and sterile jelly jars, cover well; label.

4. Store in a cool, dry place.

Tender Skin Shaving Cream

This shaving cream makes your skin luxuriantly pampered with this recipe. It's a great alternative for those with skins that are sensitive.

Ingredients

4 tablespoons solid shea butter

3 tablespoons coconut oil

2 tablespoons sweet almond oil

10-12 drops pure lavender essential oil, if desired

Instructions

1. Mix coconut oil and shea butter together

2. Transfer into a double boiler over very low heat and melt.

3. Stir from time to time. Take mixture off heat once mixture has melts totally.

4. Measure in lavender oil and almond and stir to incorporate oils well.

5. Pour mixture into a bowl and refrigerate to allow mixture solidify.

6. Whip shaving cream mixture using an electric mixer or a stand mixer.

7. Set whipped mixture aside before you transfer in a well covered jar or container.

TIP: Do not use beyond a month.

Tub Tea Treat
Ingredients

Makes: approx. 9 teabags

   2 cups Epsom salts

   15-20 drops lavender essential oil

   2 full tbsp lavender, dried

   1 cup powdered milk

   1 cup oatmeal

Instructions

1. In a large mixing bowl, combine lavender essential oil, dried lavender and Epsom salts together.

2. Mix in powdered milk into the mixing bowl mixture.

3. Use a blender or food processor, grind oatmeal to coarse powder.

4. Measure in ground oatmeal into mixing bowl.

5. Stir to combine mixing bowl mixture until well mixed.

6. Using a spoon, transfer mixture into 9 Jumbo-sized (size 4) tea filters.

7. Fold teabags at the top a few times and string tea bags.

8. Apply, one tea bag to a warm bath.

Silky Grapefruit Scrub

This out of this world grapefruit scrub leaves your skin with a beautiful and sweet fragrance. It moisturizes your skin and leaves it silky smooth.

Ingredients

Makes: 4-5 (4 ounce) Jelly jars

   1 cup coconut oil

   3-4 tablespoons grapefruit juice

   ½ cup sugar

   4-5 (4 ounce) Jelly jars

   3 tablespoons grapefruit zest, if desired

Instructions

1. Grate grapefruit zest, using a grater.

2. Mix coconut oil, zest, grapefruit juice and sugar in a medium-sized mixing bowl.

3. Stir to combine mixing bowl mixture until well combined.

4. Transfer mixture into the jars.

5. Cover and label jars.

6. Store in a well covered jar and in a cool, dry place.

NOTE: Stir if any separation occurs before use. It will stay approximately half a year.

Eucalyptus Shaving Cream

Ingredients

Makes: 2 cups

   1/2 (4 ounce) cup of coconut oil

   1/4 cup olive oil

   1/2 (4 ounce) cup shea butter

   20-25 drops eucalyptus essential oil

Instructions

1. Combine shea butter and coconut oil in a mixing bowl.

2. Transfer bowl mixture into a double boiler over medium low heat and melt.

3. Once melted, take off from heat and transfer to a bowl.

4. Measure olive oil into the mixture and stir to incorporate.

5. Refrigerate until mixture solidifies.

6. Remove from the refrigerator.

7. Using a hand mixer or standing mixer, whip bowl's mixture until stiff peaks are formed, for 3 minutes.

8. Meanwhile, as you whip mixture, measure in the essential oils.

9. Transfer whipped shaving cream into a well covered jar and store.

Concentrated Blemish/Spot Eraser Treatment

This Blemish eraser treatment is super concentrated and should be applied to spots and blemishes directly, and not your entire body or face.

Ingredients

½ tsp organic tea tree oil

5 ml glass roller bottle

4 drops lavender essential oil

½ tsp organic tamanu oil

Instructions

1. In a glass bottle, combine tea tree oil, lavender essential oil and tamanu oil together.

2. Shake to combine glass bottle mixture.

3. Apply glass roller bottle mixture to the affected skin area.

NOTE: If applied to the face to get rid of spots and blemishes; few minutes after application, wash face and apply face oil or moisturizer.

Natural Homemade Body Salt Scrub

Preparation Time: 2 minutes

Total Time: 2 minutes

Ingredients

Makes: 1 pint-sized salt scrub jar

   2 cups Epsom salt

   10-15 drops Lavender essential oil

   1 cup organic extra-virgin coconut oil

   Sprig of fresh rosemary, if desired

Instructions

1. Combine Epsom salt, lavender essential oil, rosemary and coconut oil into a large bowl.

2. Stir to combine well.

3. Pour into a mason jar and lock the cover in place.

Body Pampering Night Cream

Ingredients

    1/4 cup olive oil

    1 tablespoon Argan oil

    1 1/2 teaspoon raw honey

    1/2 teaspoon vitamin E oil

    1 teaspoon beeswax

    5 drops frankincense

    5 drops lavender essential oil

    4 ounce mason jar.

Instructions

1. Get a bowl that can withstand heat,

2. Toss in tiny pieces of beeswax and argan oil together in the bowl.

3. Heat until melted, as you stir frequently.

4. Set aside to cool for 2 to 3 minutes.

5. Mix in frankincense, lavender and vitamin E into the beeswax bowl.

6. Pour mixture into jar and cover well.

7. Store in a cool, dry place. Cream would stay 3 to 4 months.

NOTE: If due to extreme temperatures it liquefies, just refrigerate for a while.

8. Place 2 of your fingers on top of the cream and then apply to skin area.

HERBAL, ORGANIC AND ESSENTIAL OIL ANTI AGING & SKIN FIRMING RECIPES

It is possible to defy natural laws on aging. It is also possible to use natural, organic and homemade treatment to firm that skin up and look beautifully younger without visiting a plastic surgeon and using expensive cosmetics that go a long way to damage the body than help out.

Cypress Anti Aging Moisturizing Serum

This serum is quick, easy and a great recipe that will firm your skin, moisturize and add that needed glow to your skin.

Ingredients

2 tablespoons Rosehip Seed Oil

10 drops of Cypress essential oil

2 tablespoons Sweet Almond Oil

7 drops of Frankincense Essential Oil

10 drops of Geranium essential oil

2 oz glass bottle

Instructions

1. Combine rosehip seed oil, cypress essential oil, sweet almond oil, frankincense essential oil and geranium essential oil together.

2. Transfer mixture into the glass bottle.

3. Shake well to combine well.

4. Apply once or twice daily.

NOTE: Less is more, apply a little at a time, just to cover your neck and face.

Fresh Honey/Avocado Moisturizer

Ingredients

3 tbsps of fresh cream

1 tbsp honey

1/4 avocado

Instructions

1. In an electric blender, combine avocado, honey and fresh cream.

2. Blend the contents of the blender until a smooth consistency is reached.

3. Rub on the skin and allow drying for 1 hour before washing off with water.

Blood Circulating Salad

The ingredients in this recipe have antioxidant properties that keep the skin from being damaged by the sun and help the blood circulate well. This ensures that the nutrient the skin needs is adequately circulated. Recipe is to be eaten and eliminates wrinkles.

Ingredients

   1/2 cup fresh blueberries

   1 kiwi, peeled and chopped

   1/2 cup strawberries

   1/2 cup organic orange juice

   1/2 cup pomegranate seeds

   1 handful walnuts, chopped

Instructions

1. In a small bowl, combine blueberries, chopped kiwi, strawberries, and pomegranate seeds together.

2. Toss orange juice over blueberries mixture.

3. Sprinkle salad with walnuts. Serve, eat and enjoy.

Daily Anti Aging Toner

Ingredients

1 cup water

3 tbsps dried basil leaves

Instructions

1. Bring water to boiling in a pot

2. Toss crushed dried basil leaves into the hot water.

3. Using cheesecloth, strain water from the leaves.

4. Transfer into a spray bottle and apply to your skin.

NOTE: Make sure the toner is circulated on your face, using a cotton pad or ball.

Do this once a daily before cleansing your face.

Agave/Lemon Age Spot Fighter Scrub

Ingredients

1/2 cup rice, cooked

1 tbsp lemon juice

1 tbsp agave nectar

Instructions

1. Combine cooked rice, lemon juice and agave nectar together.

2. Blend together.

3. Apply a little scrub to your palm; make sure your palms are dry.

4. Use your other finger to move the scrub around in your palm in circular motions.

5. Rub this rice scrubs on callused hands and palms to soften.

NOTE: Rub firmly for 1-2 minutes with gentle pressure.

Sugar/Almond Anti Aging Face Scrub

Ingredients

3 tbsps fresh cream

1/2 cup brown sugar

1 cup white sugar

2 tbsps olive oil

1/2 cup ground almonds

Instructions

1. Combine, fresh cream, brown sugar, white sugar, olive oil and ground almonds in a small mixing bowl.

2. Mix until well combined.

3. Use your hands while applying to your face in a circular motion.

4. Using warm water, rinse your face off

5. Transfer remaining recipe into a mason jar and keep refrigerated.

Anti Aging Coconut Deep Conditioner

Ingredients

1/2 cup mayonnaise

1 tsp coconut extract

1 tbsp coconut oil

Instructions

1. Combine all the ingredients into a small bowl.

2. Stir to combine well.

3. Apply deep conditioner on hair and cover your scalp.

NOTE: Any plastic wrap would do.

4. Allow to stay on for 20-30 minutes.

5. Rinse hair with water.

NOTE: Apply once a week.

Anti Aging Lip Exfoliator

Ingredients

1/2 tsp moisturizing lotion

1/4 tsp Kosher salt

1/4 tsp fresh coffee grounds

Instructions

1. Combine moisturizing lotion, kosher salt and coffee grounds in a small bowl.

2. Rub on your mouth area completely and massage mouth area for 5 minutes.

3. Wipe your mouth clean with a wet and warm towel or wash cloth.

Rice Milk Cleanser

This recipe is known for its popularity among Japanese elites and royalty. It helps to smoothen your skin and exfoliate it.

Ingredients

2–3 tablespoons unsweetened organic rice milk

¼ cup brown rice flour (or rice bran flour)

Instructions

1. Combine rice milk and rice flour together.

2. Stir together until a fine paste consistency is reached.

3. Apply by massaging the cleanser on your skin.

NOTE: Application, should be tender and in circles.

4. Rinse with warm water and apply toner and moisturizer.

Skin Rejuvenating Cream

As you grow older, your skin dulls and dries simultaneously. This cream will help bring life and rejuvenate your skin once again; brightening your skin and returning the glory of your youth.

Ingredients

½ cup plain organic Greek yogurt

¼ cup peeled and chopped aloe flesh

¼ cup seeded and chopped cucumber

½ (juiced) lemon

Instructions

1. Combine yogurt, aloe flesh, cucumber and lemon together in a mixing bowl.

2. Blend bowl's content together in a food processor or electric blender.

3. Pulse until a smooth consistency is reached.

4. Place a mesh strainer lined with some layers cheese cloth over a bowl, then strain blenders content.

5. Strain over the night, covered.

6. In another bowl, pour the cream.

7. Apply cream generously to your face and let be for 30 minutes.

8. Wash off with a wet washcloth and apply toner.

TIP: On the flip side, the strained liquid remaining can be mixed with almond meal/rice flour, for a very effective face scrub.

Blueberry Granola Anti Aging Exfoliating Mask

Ingredients

¼ cup fresh organic blueberries

¼ cup raw almonds

2 tablespoons whole oats

1 tablespoon honey

1 tablespoon whole organic milk

Instructions

1. Mix blueberries, whole oats, almonds, organic milk and honey together into a small bowl.

2. Transfer bowl mixture into food processor or an electric blender.

3. Blend until a fine consistency is reached.

NOTE: While blending, you can add more milk, for required consistency.

4. Moisten your skin, and then apply richly to the skin.

5. Leave for 20 minutes to dry.

6. Rinse with warm water and apply your toner.

Age Spots Reduction Oil

Ingredients

Few drops frankincense oil

Instructions

1. Apply few drops of frankincense oil to your skin directly.

2. Do this three times a day to improve and gradually correct age spots and sun spots.

Anti Aging Skin Scrub

Ingredients

½ cup fresh organic blackberries

½ cup walnuts

Instructions

1. Place all ingredients together in a small bowl.

2. Transfer bowl mixture into a food processor or electric blender.

3. Blend until a smooth consistency is reached.

4. Moisten your skin, and then apply paste richly to the skin.

5. Massage skin area in circular motions.

6. Rinse with warm water and apply your toner and cleanser.

NOTE: If you don't have blackberries around, you can use black raspberries as a substitute.

Avocado Wheatgrass Anti Aging Mask
This anti aging recipe helps to renew the texture of the skin and also fights damage from aging-causing free radicals.

Ingredients

½ ripe avocado

1 tablespoon wheatgrass juice

2 tablespoon plain organic Greek yogurt

Instructions

1. Place all ingredients together in a small bowl.

2. Transfer bowl mixture into a food processor or electric blender.

3. Blend until a smooth consistency is reached.

4. Moisten your skin, and then apply paste richly to your skin.

5. Leave for 15 to 20 minutes to dry.

6. Rinse with warm water and apply your toner.

Honeyed Anti Aging Scrub

Ingredients

½ cup raw green apple, chopped

2 tablespoons chia seeds

2 tablespoons honey

Instructions

1. Place all ingredients together in a small bowl.

2. Transfer bowl mixture into a food processor or electric blender.

3. Blend until a smooth consistency is reached.

NOTE: Add water where necessary.

4. Set aside for 5 minutes.

5. Moisten your skin, and then apply paste richly to your skin.

6. Massage skin area in gentle and not too fast circular motions.

7. Rinse with warm water and apply your toner.

Body Anti Aging Oil

Ingredients

¼ cup avocado oil

¼ cup melted coconut oil

¼ cup sweet almond oil

8 oz. bottle

Instructions

1. Place all ingredients together in a small bottle.

2. Shake vigorously to combine.

3. Rub on the body every day, from your shoulders to your toes.

4. Massaging the oils in.

Eye Anti Aging Roll On

Ingredients

1 tablespoon meadowfoam seed oil

1 1/2 teaspoon beeswax

2 teaspoons unrefined organic coconut oil

1/2 teaspoon Vitamin E oil

1/2 teaspoon shea butter

5 drops frankincense essential oil

4 drops carrot seed essential oil

8 drops lavender essential oil

Instructions

1. In a double boiler over low heat, measure coconut oil, meadowfoam seed oil, shea butter and beeswax in.

2. Take off from heat once shea butter mixture melts completely.

3. Measure in vitamin E oil, frankincense, carrot seed and lavender essential oils into the mixture.

4. Transfer into a lip balm tube.

Green Tea Anti Aging Cream

This recipe is an anti aging recipe and also firms the eye

Ingredients

Makes: 4 ounces

1/4 cup green tea

1 tablespoon rosehip seed oil

1/8 teaspoon NeoDefend

1/4 teaspoon vitamin E

1 tablespoon sweet almond oil

1 drop carrot Seed essential Oil

1 teaspoon emulsifying wax

3 drops lavender Essential Oil

Instructions

1. Fill 2 medium sized sauce pans half way with water.

2. On medium heat, place 1 glass bowl that has a spout into each sauce pan.

3. Measure in rosehip seed oil, wax, sweet almond oil and vit.E oil into one of the glass bowl inside the sauce pan.

TIP: Meanwhile before step 1, brew one cup of green tea

4. Measure in NeoDefend and the brewed green tea into the second glass bowl in the other sauce pan.

5. Heat the mixtures in the two separate sauce pans until the wax melts completely.

7. Take the temperatures of the two sauce pans with a thermometer.

NOTE: Both have to be at same for the cream to set when combined. Otherwise your cream would not set.

8. When both mixtures in the saucepan reach 130°F, pour the green tea mixture into the rosehip seed oil mixture.

9. Combine cream together, using a hand blender.

10. Mix every ten minutes thereabout for 30-60 minutes, until water doesn't separate at the bottom anymore

11. Measure in essential oils into the mixture once it is fully mixed.

12. This cream works well under make up, use morning and night.

Daily Anti Aging Eye Cream

This recipe helps to restore youth, remove wrinkles and lines.

Ingredients

1/2 cup Organic coconut oil

10 drops frankincense essential Oil

6-8 Vitamin E capsules

Instructions

1. Place a saucepan over low heat.

2. Measure in coconut oil into the saucepan and melt for some minutes until completely melted.

3. Transfer melted coconut oil into a clean container with cover.

4. Pierce the vitamin E capsules and squeeze oil into the coconut oil container.

5. Stir to incorporate.

6. Measure in the essential oil.

7. Refrigerate for 30-60 minutes until the mixture solidifies.

NOTE: Once it solidifies, you don't need to refrigerate anymore.

8. Dab a little quantity of cream beneath your eyes at once at night and occasionally in the morning.

Homemade Facial Cream

This facial cream recipe is a helps to tighten the face and rejuvenate the skin

Ingredients

Makes: approx. ½ cup

¼ cup almond oil

2 tbsps beeswax

2 tbsps coconut oil

1 tbsp shea butter

½ tsp vitamin E oil

Any of your favorite essential oils, if desired

Instructions

1. Combine almond oil, beeswax, coconut oil, and shea butter together.

2. Melt in a double boiler over low heat. Stir from time to time.

3. Take off from heat and set aside, once melted.

4. Add your favorite essential oil(s) and vitamin E oil.

5. Stir to incorporate.

6 Transfer into a glass jar, set aside until mixture solidifies.

7. Cover and store in a cool, dry place.

8. Apply twice daily, morning and night after face wash.

NOTE: Cream will stay for as long as 3 months.

Hi-C Face Healing Serum

This rich in natural vitamin C facial serum destroys wrinkles and reverses damage to the skin. It is also used to strengthen the barrier response of the skin, build collagen, reduce inflammation and many more.

Ingredients

1/4 cup aloe vera gel

2 teaspoons natural vitamin c powder

1 tablespoon fresh hibiscus petals or 1/2 tablespoon dried Hibiscus flowers

1/4 teaspoons vitamin E, if desired

Instructions

1. Mix dried hibiscus with aloe gel together.

2. Transfer aloe gel mixture into an electric blender or food processor.

3. Blend until the hibiscus changes to a pink-like color, for 5 to 10 times.

4. Set aside to extract favorable flavors, for 30 minutes.

5. Use a cloth/mesh strainer, strain aloe gel by squeezing it out from the hibiscus.

NOTE: You can straight twice, just to make sure you strained well.

6. Mix in vitamin C into the mixture slowly into the aloe vera gel mixture.

7. Stir well until natural vitamin C powder is well incorporated into the mixture.

8. Transfer into a dark bottle and lock lid in place.

NOTE: The dark bottle helps to keep the sun out, and preserve the longevity of vitamin C in the recipe.

9. Refrigerate bottle.

10. After toning and cleansing your face apply the serum to your décolleté, neck and face. Then moisturize your face.

NOTE: The vitamin E is a good combination with Vitamin C, and it also prevents the vitamin C in the recipe, from oxidizing so fast.

Bentonite Cocoa Mud Mask

This mud mask energizes

Preparation Time: 2 minutes

Cook Time: 15 minutes

Ingredients

1 tbsp cocoa powder

1 tsp coffee, finely ground

1 tbsp Bentonite clay

Few tsps of water

Instructions

1. In a plastic bowl, Toss in the cocoa powder, ground coffee and bentonite clay.

2. Toss in sufficient water for a fine paste.

3. Using a wooden spoon stir mixture together until a paste-like consistency has been reached.

NOTE: Make sure you make use of a wooden spoon and a plastic bowl. Metals are not allowed with this recipe.

4. Apply using clean hands to rub on your chest and the face.

5. Allow mud mask to stay and dry for 15 minutes after application to the skin area.

6. Wash mask off, and then massage coffee into your skin, gently to exfoliate.

Rosehip Décolleté Neck & Face Serum

Ingredient

2 tablespoons rosehip seed oil

10 drops of cypress essential oil

2 tablespoons sweet almond oil

7 drops of frankincense essential oil

10 drops of geranium essential oil

2 oz. glass bottle.

Instructions

1. Combine rosehip seed oil, cypress essential oil, sweet almond oil, frankincense essential oil, and geranium essential oil.

2. Stir till a fine consistency is reached.

3. Transfer into a glass bottle.

4. Shake vigorously before use twice daily.

NOTE: Just a little amount just to cover your face and neck.

HERBAL, ORGANIC AND ESSENTIAL OIL RECIPES TO FIGHT ACNE, BLEMISHES AND SPOTS

Your skin is in love with you and you are in love with your skin. Your skin is a loyal friend and you are a proud friend to your skin also. This beautiful relationship goes on for a while...

One day you wake up to discover that acne appears and damages the cordial relationship you have built with your skin over time.

Suddenly you start to hate and resent your skin. What is the next line of action? How can this love and friendship be restored?

It is not farfetched! The answer is not in harsh store bought chemicals. Simple answer... GO ORGANIC!

You will get maximum results if you start treating and handling your skin the right way.

ACV Clay Mask

Ingredients

- 2 tbsps apple cider vinegar

- 2 tbsps bentonite clay

Instructions

1. Combine ingredients well until thoroughly mixed.

NOTE: When well mixed, the mask will become thick

2. Avoid your eye area when applying to the face.

3. Leave on the face to dry for 10 to 20 minutes.

NOTE: If you have a skin that is sensitive, leave it for approximately 10 minutes.

Vinegar-Water Anti-Acne Recipe

A bacteria killer, it eliminates acne causing bacteria and the pH of your skin gets balanced also; an astringent known to dry out too much oil on the skin.

Ingredients

3 tbsps fresh water

1 tbsp apple cider vinegar (pure & unfiltered)

Instructions

1. In a small bowl, combine water and apple cider vinegar together.

2. Mix well.

3. Wash your face well.

4. Place a cotton ball into the mixture gently, and apply vinegar soaked cotton ball on affected skin area, blemishes and acne.

5. Leave on your face 10 minutes before washing off thoroughly.

NOTE: You can leave it over the night and can be reapplied anytime in the day; this can be done many times.

6. After you wash off, moisturize your face.

Yogurt-y Spot Removal Mask

Ingredients

> 1 tbsp honey (raw & natural)

> 1 tbsp yogurt or milk (plain low-fat or full-fat)

Instructions

1. Set refrigerated milk or yogurt aside to cool properly.

2. Combine yogurt/milk with honey in a small bowl.

3. Mix thoroughly until well combined.

4. Wash your face and pat dry.

5. Apply by patting a thick layer of the mask on your face.

NOTE: For desired thickness, allow first layer dry before adding another layer. Repeat process until desired thickness is reached.

6. Leave on for 10 to 15 minutes to dry.

7. Wash your face, dry gently with a wash cloth to get rid of dead skin that has been loosened.

8. Apply moisturizer.

NOTE: You can use any plain full fat or low fat yogurt or milk, but do not use anything skimmed.

Honey with Cinnamon Face Mask

Ingredients

1 tsp cinnamon

2 tbsps honey

Instructions

1. Combine cinnamon and honey together in a bowl.

2. Mix together until well combined.

NOTE: A paste-like consistency should be reached.

3. Wash your face well, pat dry and apply mask to your face or area affected with spots.

4. Leave on for 10 to 15 minutes.

5. Wash face thoroughly and dry your face.

Acne Aromatherapy Oil

Ingredients

1 oz.fl., Jojoba or Fractionated Coconut Oil

5 drops Tea Tree Oil

6 drops Lavender Oil

1 drop Geranium Oil

Instructions

1. In a well cleaned amber glass bottle, measure in Jojoba or fractionated coconut oil.

2. Measure in tea tree oil, lavender oil and Geranium oil into the glass bottle.

NOTE: Undiluted essential oils shouldn't be stored in bottles with rubber tops. It is okay to store this recipe in a dropper top bottle, because it has been well diluted.

3. Gently mix the bottle's content by rolling the bottle for 1-2 minutes.

4. Avoid application of recipe to the lips, eyes, inside the ears and nostrils. Limit application of recipe to the face, back and neck in small amounts.

Honeyed tea tree Anti-Acne Face Wash

Ingredients

Raw honey

Tea tree oil

Instructions

1. Combine raw honey and tea tree oil together.

2. Apply to your face to rid your face of acne.

3. Rinse your face off with water.

Papaya Anti-Acne Paste

Ingredient

1 papaya, fresh

Instructions

1. Using a mortar and pestle or an electric blender, blend or grind the papaya flesh well adding a very small amount of water to form a paste.

NOTE: Add little water at a time, so as not to flood your mixture.

2. Keep blending until a paste-like consistency is reached.

3. Wash your face and pat dry.

4. Apply a thick layer to the affected areas or your face.

5. Leave on your face for 15 to 20 minutes.

6. Wash off from face and dry your face.

7. Apply moisturizer.

Egg whites Scar fading Mask

A simple and purse friendly way to remove scars and fight acne

Ingredients

Washcloth

2 -3 egg whites (yolks removed)

Bowl

Instructions

1. Boil eggs until well cooked.

2. Set aside to cool, and then peel.

3. Remove yolks from egg whites.

4. Whisk egg whites until a frothy consistency is reached.

5. Set aside for 2-3 minutes.

6. Wash your face and pat dry.

7. Apply a thick layer of the mask to the affected area/spot/scar with the tips of your fingers.

NOTE: a) Clean your hands before application. b) Apply in succession, first layer dries out first before adding another layer. 3-4 layers should be okay for thick layer.

8. Leave on for 20 minutes to dry.

9. Wash face off, using warm water, and pat dry.

10 Moisturize your face accordingly.

Tea Tree Oil Remedy

This remedy works a natural magic that cuts through oily skin and skin cells that are dead and opens up the pores. Kills acne causing bacteria and prevents a reoccurrence.

Ingredients

1 tbsp tea tree oil

Cotton balls

9 tbsps Water, clean and fresh

Instructions

1. Combine water and tea tree oil together in a bowl.

2. Mix together until well combined.

3. Wash your face well, pat dry and apply remedy to your face or area affected with spots slowly, using cotton balls.

4. Apply moisturizer after application.

NOTE: a) You can make your mix stronger by changing the ratio of tea tree oil to water slightly. But don't start in a rush; change preparation ratio slightly only after having used this mixture's ratio consistently for a minimum of a week. b) Aloe vera gel can be used as a substitute for water.

Orange Peel Paste Mask

Ingredients

2 Orange peels

Water, fresh and clean

Instructions

1. Using a mortar and pestle or an electric blender, blend or grind the orange peels adding a small amount of water to form a paste.

NOTE: Add little water at a time, so as not to flood your mixture.

2. Keep blending until a paste-like consistency is reached.

3. Wash your face and pat dry.

4. Apply a thick layer to the affected areas or your face.

5. Leave on your face for 20 to 25 minutes.

6. Wash off from face and dry your face.

7. Apply moisturizer.

Banana Peel Face Healing

Ingredients

   1 banana peel

Instructions

1. Separate peels from banana.

2. Apply by rubbing peels in circular motions over your face.

3. Leave on face for 30 minutes.

4. Wash off.

Honey & Strawberries Mix

Ingredients

   2 tsps of raw honey

   3 clean & fresh strawberries

   Clean water

Instructions

1. Wash Strawberries and make sure they are clean.

2. Grind/pound strawberries well, adding very few drops of water.

NOTE: Don't over pound

3. Combine honey and mashed strawberries together.

4. Mix thoroughly until well combined.

5. Wash your face and pat dry.

6. Apply a thick layer to the affected areas or your face.

7. Leave on your face for 20 minutes.

6. Wash off from face with warm water and dry your face.

NOTE: Use 2 times weekly for 1 month or more.

Face Exfoliating Mask

Baking soda also known as Sodium bicarbonate is known to exfoliate the skin, fight off bacteria and fungus, and also help to dry off excess skin oil. Your skin becomes glamorous and tender.

Ingredients

Fresh water

1 box baking soda

Instructions

1. Combine same amounts of water and baking soda together.

2. Stir to combine until a paste-like consistency is reached.

3. Wash face and pat dry.

4. Apply by massaging baking soda mask on your face and affected areas for 2 minutes. Move in circles as you apply.

5. Allow to dry for 15 to 20 minutes before washing off and pat drying gently.

NOTE: Use warm water to wash off.

6. Apply moisturizer.

Aloe Gel Anti-Acne Remedy

Ingredients

Aloe vera gel

Instructions

1. Wash and pat dry your face.

2. Apply a thick layer of aloe gel to the spot and other affected areas or your face.

3. Leave on your face for 10 minutes.

4. Wash off from face with warm water and dry your face.

Lemon Juice Touch

Ingredients

1 tbsp lemon juice, just squeezed

Yogurt, if desired

Cotton balls, if desired

Instructions

1. Combine yogurt and lemon juice together.

2. Stir to combine until well mixed.

3. Wash face and pat dry.

4. Apply by dipping cotton balls into yogurt/lemon mixture and rub on acne and other affected skin areas.

5. Wash off and pat dry gently.

NOTE: Use warm water to wash off.

Face Clearing Massage Scrub

Ingredients

1/8 cup fresh water

1/2 cup baking soda

Instructions

1. Combine water and baking soda together.

2. Stir to combine until a paste-like consistency is reached.

3. Wash face and pat dry.

4. Apply by massaging in the baking soda mask into your face and affected areas for 5 to 6 minutes.

NOTE: Move in circles as you apply.

5. Wash off and pat dry gently.

NOTE: Use warm water to wash off.

6. Apply moisturizer.

Garlic Natural Remedy

Ingredients

Aloe vera gel

2-3 cloves of garlic

Instructions

1. Pound the cloves of garlic until well mashed.

2. Measure in the aloe vera gel. Set aside to soak for 10 minutes.

3. Mash well until well mixed.

4. Dip cotton pad into the garlic juice and apply to spots/blemishes and acnes.

TIP: You can use remedy daily.

Steam Face & Beauty Routine Treatment

Steam helps to open up the skin and remove dirt, impurity that is beneath the skin. Steam alone works fine, but you can use this treatment before applying some other organic beauty treatments. The steam helps to clear the way for the other beauty treatments or recipes to do this its work effectively.

Ingredients

1 pot water

1 towel

1 large bowl

Instructions

1. Bring a pot of water to boiling.

2. Transfer water into the bowl.

3. Set aside for few minutes to lose a little bit of heat.

4. Set your face above the bowl, stopping short a little distance from the bowl.

5. To trap the steam and get maximum results; with the towel, cover your head, neck region and the bowl together.

NOTE: Drape towel in such a way that you contain as much of the steam as possible within the towel confinement.

6. Continue treatment for 10 to 15 minutes before pat drying your face.

TIP: You can do this every night or every morning or as needed.

Sugar Anti-Acne Fighting Scrub
Ingredients

Makes: 4 half pint jars

1 ½ cups white sugar

2-3 tbsps coarse sea salt

1 ½ cups (light or dark) brown sugar

10 tbsps pure vanilla extract

1/2 cup (approx.) olive oil

1 whole vanilla bean, if desired, (with caviar scrapped out)

Instructions

1. Combine white sugar, coarse sea salt, brown sugar and vanilla bean together.

2. Mix mixture thoroughly

3. In a liquid measuring cup, measure out two cups of this sugar/salt mixture.

NOTE: Press the mixture down to fill all air spaces in the measuring cup.

4. Toss olive oil over the measuring cup mixture and let it be absorbed by half the mixture.

5. Leave small layer on the top and spoon in 4 or 5 tbsps of vanilla extract into the mixture and stir to combine.

6. Transfer into smaller jars for use.

Honeyed Oatmeal Booster

Ingredients

1 serving of oatmeal

2 tbsps honey, raw

Water

Instructions

1. Follow preparation instructions on the box of oatmeal; prepare oatmeal.

2. Take off from heat.

3. Measure in the honey.

4. Stir to incorporate honey into oatmeal well.

5. Set aside to cool to room temperature.

NOTE: Be sure it has really cooled.

6. Apply on skin and leave for 20 to 30 minutes to dry.

7 Wash off with warm water and pat dry.

Mint Fresh Facial Mask

Ingredients

1 heaping handful of mint leaves, fresh

Instructions

1. In an electric blender, blend fresh mint leaves.

2. Blend until well mashed up.

3. Wash face and pat dry.

4. Apply crushed mint juice and leaves on your face.

5. Leave on for 5 to 10 minutes before washing with cold water.

6. Pat dry.

Honey & Avocado Paste

Ingredients

1 tbsp of honey

1 avocado

Instructions

1. Remove the inside part of the avocado and pound it.

2. Stir mashed avocado inside with honey.

3. Keep pounding and stirring until a paste-like consistency is reached.

4. Wash your face and pat dry.

5. Apply honey and avocado face mask to your face.

6. Leave on 15 to 20 minutes.

7. Wash off with warm water and pat dry gently.

8. Moisturize your skin.

Mashed Potato Face Mask

Ingredients

1 potato, raw

Instructions

1. In a grater, grate potato.

2. Grate until well mashed up.

3. Wash face and pat face until almost dry.

4. Apply juice and pulp onto your face; moving in circles as you apply.

5. Leave on for 15 to 30 minutes to dry.

6. Wash off with warm water.

7. Pat dry.

Acne Spot & Blemish Treatment

Ingredients

Brewer's yeast

Few tsps of water

1 squeeze of lemon juice

Instructions

1. Combine yeast, water and lemon juice together.

2. Mix to combine until paste-like consistency is reached.

3. Wash face and pat dry.

4. Apply the paste directly on your spots or blemishes.

5. Leave on for 8 to 10 minutes and covering with a bandage.

Face Oil Reducing Tea

Recipe decreases skin oil, skin bacteria and inflammation. For topical use and can also be ingested to detoxify the body.

Ingredients

1 green tea bag or 2 tsps loose organic tea leaves

1/2 cup fresh water

Instructions

1. Bring water to a boil in a pot over medium heat.

2. Place tea leaves or tea bags in a bowl and pour the hot water on it.

3. Set aside for 4 to 5 minutes to release tea flavors.

4. Using mesh strainer or cheesecloth, strain out the leaves and set aside tea liquid to cool.

5. Transfer into a glass spray bottle and apply to your face lightly.

TIP: You can rinse off if you want to, and you can also leave on.

HERBAL, ORGANIC AND ESSENTIAL OIL SEA SALT TREATMENT RECIPES

Skin Balancing Mask

Corrects irritation and breakouts, soothes and calms the skin. Helps to balance skin oil production also

Ingredients

2 tsps finely ground sea salt

4 tsps honey, raw

Instructions

1. Combine honey and salt together in a small bowl.

2. Stir well to combine until a paste like consistency is reached.

3. Wash and pat dry skin.

4. Apply to the skin.

NOTE: Do not make mistakes of applying on the eyes.

5. Leave on for 10-15 minutes before washing with warm water.

TIP: a) Before washing your face, use a warm washcloth on your face; to massage your face for 30 seconds. b) Move your hands in circular movements.

Tender Body Salt Scrub

Ingredients

1/4 cup salt

10 drops of your favorite essential oil

1/2 cup softened coconut oil or olive oil

Instructions

1. Combine salt and oil together

2. Stir well until a thick paste-like consistency is reached.

3. Measure in the essential of your choosing and stir to incorporate.

4. Wash face and pat dry.

5. Apply using a wash cloth or your palms to tenderly scrub your skin moving in circles.

Oil Removing Sea Salt Facial Toner

This facial toner helps to clean pores and drastically reduce oil production and fight bacteria.

Ingredients

1 tsp sea salt

4 oz. clean water.

Instructions

1. Bring water to boiling and set aside until warm.

2. Combine warm water and salt together.

3. Mix until the salt dissolves.

4. Transfer into a spray bottle.

5. Spritz on your face.

Warm Salt Bath

This salt bath helps to relax the body

Ingredients

1/3 cup salt

1 full tub of warm water.

Instructions

1. Swish sea salt into the bath tub filled with warm water to dissolve.

2. Soak for 15-30 minutes.

Aloe Gel Salt Scrub

Ingredients

1/2 cup salt

1/4 cup olive oil

1/4 cup aloe vera gel

1 tbsps of lavender flowers, dried.

Instructions

1. Combine salt, oil and aloe vera gel together.

2. Mix until a thick paste-like consistency is reached.

NOTE: if mixture is too dry, add little oil more.

3. Wash face and pat dry.

4. Apply using a wash cloth or your palms to tenderly scrub your skin moving in circles.

Teeth Whitening Powder

Ingredients

2 tsps baking powder

1 tsp salt

Instructions

1. Combine baking powder and salt together.

2. Mix until properly combined.

3. Wet toothbrush with water and dip into baking powder mixture.

4. Apply brushing your teeth as you would with regular toothpaste.

TIP: You can add a little bit of your regular toothpaste with this mixture.

Anti-Dandruff Salt Treatment

This recipe combats fungi and absorbs excessive moisture on the skin and the scalp.

Ingredients

1-2 tsps salt.

Few drops of water

Instructions

1. Apply by sprinkling salt on your scalp.

2. Moisten your hands with water and massage scalp thoroughly with wet hands for 10-15 minutes.

3. Wash, pat dry your hair. Apply hair conditioning cream.

Nail Brightening Salt/Warm Water Solution

Ingredients

1 tsp salt

1 tsp baking soda

1 tsp lemon juice

1/2 cup water

Instructions

1. Warm water in a small pot.

2. In a small bowl, combine salt, lemon juice, warm water and baking soda together.

3. Dip your nails into the warm water salt solution for 10 minutes.

4. After 10 minutes, your nails should be scrubbed using soft brush.

5. Rinse your hands and apply moisturizer.

Salt Soda Mouth Wash

Ingredients

    1/2 tsp salt

    1/2 tsp baking soda

    1/4 cup water

Instructions

1. Combine baking soda, salt and water together.

2. Mix well until the salt is dissolved in the mixture.

3. Pour a little of the solution into your mouth, swish around and gargle.

4. Spit out and then wash your mouth.

HERBAL, ORGANIC AND ESSENTIAL OIL SKIN CLEARING RECIPES

Honeyed Lemon Mix

This honeyed lemon mix clears the skin and brightens your skin tone

Ingredients

Freshly squeezed lemon juice

1-2 tbsps honey, raw

Instructions

1. Extract juice from lemon.

2. Combine honey and lemon juice. Stir until consistent.

3. Wash face and pat dry.

4. Apply to the neck region and the face.

5. Leave on for 15-20 minutes.

6. Wash off with warm water and pat face dry.

7. Rub slices of cucumber on your skin to moisturize and soften your skin.

TIP: You can give your skin this treat daily or thrice weekly.

Honeyed Milk Skin Clearing Mix

Ingredients

2 tsps milk

1 tsp honey

1 tsp gram flour

Instructions

1. Combine milk, honey and flower together.

2. Stir together until a paste like consistency is reached.

3. Wash and pat dry face.

4. Rub on your face and leave to dry for 20 minutes.

5. Wash your face with warm water and pat dry.

TIP: Apply once weekly for a clear and bright skin.

Pine-Turmeric Mix

Ingredients

1 tbsp turmeric powder

Few tsps pineapple juice

Instructions

1. Combine turmeric and pineapple together and mix well.

2. Wash face and pat dry.

3. Apply the paste to the neck and face and leave for 15 to 20 minutes.

4. Wash with warm water and pat dry.

TIP: Use 2-3 times weekly.

Lemon Soda Skin Clearing Mix

Ingredients

1 tsp baking soda

1 tsp water

1 tsp lemon juice

Instructions

1. Combine ingredients together.

2. Mix until paste-like consistency is reached.

3. Wash your face and pat dry.

4. Apply as a mask for exfoliating the skin.

5. Leave to dry and wash off with warm water, pat dry.

TIP: Use 2-3 times weekly.

Aloe Gel Moisturizing Skin Clearing Mix

This recipe helps new skin cells to grow and moisturizes the skin

Ingredients

Aloe vera gel

Cotton ball

Instructions

1. Wash and pat dry your face.

2. Use cotton ball to apply aloe gel on your face.

3. Leave on for 30 minutes.

4. Wash off with warm water.

TIP: Once every day for 5 months.

Honeyed Papaya Mix

This treat works as a skin clearing mix, clears and brightens the skin; leaves your skin texture as a baby's

Ingredients

Ripe papaya, chopped

1 tsp sandalwood powder

1 tsp honey

Instructions

1. Combine ingredients together.

2. Blend mixture until a paste like consistency is reached.

3. Wash and pat dry your face.

4. Apply to the face and leave on for 30-60 minutes.

5. Wash off and dry.

6. Follow with rose water to the face.

TIP: This should be used once weekly for a tremendous quantifiable change in skin tone.

Lemon Cucumber Mix

Ingredients

1 tbsp of cucumber juice

1 tbsp of lemon juice

Instructions

1. Combine ingredients together.

2. Stir until well combined.

3. Wash and pat dry your skin.

4. Apply mixture to affected skin area, leave to dry; and then wash off.

TIP: Use daily.

Walnut Skin Clearing Mix

Ingredients

2 tsps walnut powder

2 tbsps plain yogurt

Instructions

1. Come both ingredients together.

2. Stir well until paste-like consistency is reached.

3. Wash and pat dry your face.

4. Apply to the face and leave on till paste dries off, for 60 minutes.

5. Wash off with warm water and dry your face by patting.

TIP: a) This should be used once weekly for a tremendous quantifiable change in skin tone.

b) Eat 2-3 walnuts with 1 glass of milk each morning. Mix two teaspoons of walnut powder with two tablespoons of plain yogurt to make a paste. Apply this paste on.

HERBAL, ORGANIC AND ESSENTIAL OIL DIY SHAMPOO HAIR TREATMENT

You can make your own shampoo and give your hair the care, treatment and pampering it deserves.

Castile Flavored Shampoo

Ingredients

¼ cup liquid Castile soap

¼ cup water

½ tsp oil (like grapeseed, olive oil or jojoba)

Instructions

1. Combine Liquid castile soap, water and any oil of your choice.

2. Mix together and combine well.

3. Transfer mixture into a plastic or glass bottle.

4. Shake well before each use.

NOTE: This combination works well for some hair types, textures and colors. For some others, they have reported that the shampoo leaves a film on their hair. The type of hair you have and the type of water used can have so much impact on the result gotten from this shampoo's use.

Simple Hair Care Shampoo
This shampoo gives a really impressive lather.

Ingredients

Foaming Bottles or Flip Cap Bottles to dispense

¼ cup of liquid Castile Soap (unscented or your favorite)

¼ cup of water (distilled)

½ tsp of grapeseed, jojoba or other light vegetable oil

Instructions

1. Combine Liquid castile soap, water and any oil of your choice.

2. Mix together and combine well.

3. Transfer mixture into a flip cap bottle.

4. Shake well before each use.

5. Apply by tilting the bottle slightly over your head.

Baking Soda with ACV Shampoo

Ingredients

3 cups water

1/2 cup baking soda

1/2 cup apple cider vinegar/ regular white vinegar

Instructions

1. Combine baking soda and warm water together.

2. Stir to combine until thoroughly mixed.

3. Transfer into a plastic or glass container.

4. Shake well before each use.

5. Apply by scrubbing shampoo into your scalp.

6. Wash off with vinegar.

TIP: You may decide to tweak ingredient ratios slightly until you find what works for you perfectly.

NOTE: It takes 2-4 weeks for your body to adjust to this new shampoo. Before now, you probably have been using store bought commercial products which have stripped your body of natural oils on a daily basis. Once you start using this natural shampoo, you hair may start to feel thick or oily as you start to gradually adjust.

Tea Mint Hair Rousing Shampoo

At some point you may want to stimulate and wake up your scalp from its sleep. The ingredients in this recipe will help make that a reality.

Ingredients

   1/8 teaspoon tea tree essential oil

   ¼ cup water (distilled)

   1/8 teaspoon peppermint essential oil

   2 teaspoon jojoba oil

   ¼ cup liquid Castile Soap (unscented or your favorite)

   Flip Cap Bottles or Foaming Bottles to dispense

Instructions

1. Combine liquid castile soap with jojoba oil together in a small mixing bowl.

2. Stir together until well combined.

3. Add the distilled water and stir well.

4. Measure in tea tree and peppermint essential oils.

5. Stir well until oils have been well distributed.

6. Transfer mixture into a flip cap bottle.

7. Shake well before each use.

8. Apply as you would any regular shampoo.

9. Wash your hair and pat dry.

Organic Lavender Shampoo
This shampoo mix corrects itchy scalp

Ingredients

Few drops lavender, basil or cedarwood essential oils

Organic shampoo

Instructions

1. Get a regular organic shampoo,

2. Toss in few drops of lavender oil, basil oil or cedarwood oil into the shampoo.

3. Apply on scalp to eliminate itching.

Homemade Lavender Rose Shampoo

Ingredients

Rosemary essential oil

Lavender essential oil

Coconut milk

Aloe vera gel

Instructions

1. Combine rosemary oil, lavender oil, coconut milk and aloe vera gel.

2. Apply to hair the same way you would a regular shampoo.

Organic Rose Shampoo
This Shampoo thickens your hair

Ingredients

Organic shampoo

Rosemary essential oil

Instructions

1. Get a regular organic shampoo,

2. Add rosemary oil to it.

3. Apply on hair to make your hair become thick naturally and increase its volume.

Lavender Ylang Ylang Shampoo

This recipe is easy to make

Ingredients

7 fluid ounces Unscented Shampoo Base

40 drops Lavender essential Oil

1 tbsp Jojoba {if desired} (gives the hair added hydration)

5 drops Ylang Ylang essential Oil

10 drops Rosemary essential Oil

Instructions

1. Get a mixing bowl,

2. Toss in the unscented shampoo base into the bowl,

3. Blend in lavender, jojoba, ylang ylang and rosemary essential oils.

4. Combine thoroughly until essential oils are well incorporated.

5. Pour shampoo into an 8 ounce bottle, using a funnel.

NOTE: Adhere to all essential oil safety precautions when using any essential oil or blend. Always do a skin patch test for essential oils before usage, make sure the essential oils you are using are gentle to the skin.

6. Apply as you would a regular shampoo.

Aloe Gel Anti-Bacterial Shampoo

This recipe is a hair growth potion that is anti-fungal and anti-bacterial

Ingredients

1/4-1/2 cup water

Aloe Vera gel (better if it's fresh)

Rosemary essential oil

Instructions

1. Combine aloe gel, water and essential oil together in a bowl.

2. Stir together and transfer into an electric blender.

3. Blend until a smooth consistency has been reached.

4. Transfer mixture into a container.

Lavender Hair Care Shampoo

Ingredients

1 ½ tbsps of glycerin

1 cup castile soap (Lavender)

1 cup of water, distilled

6 chamomile tea bags

Instructions

1. Brew a cup of chamomile tea. Bring water to boiling.

2. Transfer into a tea cup and leave chamomile tea bags in the cup for 20 minutes.

3. Measure in liquid castile soap into the tea, stirring to combine.

4. Measure in glycerin into the tea mixture and stir thoroughly until well incorporated.

5. Transfer mixture into a dark glass bottle and cover well.

6. Store in a cool, dry and dark place.

Hair Drying Shampoo Mix

Ingredients

¼ cup of distilled water

¼ cup of aloe vera gel

¼ cup of liquid Castile Soap (your favorite scent)

¼ tsp of jojoba oil or avocado oil

1 tsp of glycerin

Flip Cap Bottles or Foaming Bottles to dispense

Instructions

1. Combine aloe vera gel, liquid castile soap, avocado/jojoba oil, water, and glycerin together in a small mixing bowl.

2. Stir to combine until thoroughly mixed.

3. Transfer into a flip cap bottle.

4. Shake well before each use.

5. Apply by scrubbing shampoo into your scalp.

Natural Lemon Shampoo For A Glowing Hair

This recipe brings a radiant liveliness to your hair. It is fragrant and would add the desired and needed shine to your hair.

Ingredients

2 tablespoons of rosemary, dried

¼ cup of water, distilled

¼ cup of liquid Castile Soap (use lemon)

¼ lemon essential oil

2 tablespoons sweet almond oil

Flip Cap Bottles or Foaming Bottles to dispense

Instructions

1. Bring water to boiling in a pot over medium high heat.

2. Measure in rosemary and then leave for a while to release flavor into hot water, until water becomes fragrant.

3. Using a mesh strainer or cheesecloth, strain water from leaves and set rosemary flavored water aside to cool.

4. After cooling, measure in the liquid castile soap, sweet almond oil and lemon essential oil.

5. Stir well to combine.

6. Transfer mixture into a flip cap bottle and store in a cool, dry place.

7. Apply as you would a regular shampoo.

Hair Anti-Flake Shampoo

This shampoo is a flaky scalp remedy; it will give your scalp and hair the freshness you deserve.

Ingredients

¼ cup of water, distilled

1 tbsp of apple cider vinegar

¼ cup of liquid Castile Soap

½ tsp of grapeseed, jojoba, or other light vegetable oil

6 finely ground cloves

3 tbsps of apple juice

Flip Cap Bottles or Foaming Bottles to dispense

Instructions

1. Combine vinegar, castile soap, grapeseed oil, water, ground cloves and apple juice together in a mixing bowl.

2. Transfer mixture into an electric blender or small grinder.

3. Blend mixture together for 30 seconds.

4. Transfer mixture into flip cap bottles.

5. Warm water, and wet your hair before applying shampoo as you would a regular shampoo.

6. Wash your hair and pat dry.

7. Refrigerate remaining shampoo.

NOTE: It has a 3 day shelf life.

Lavender Hair Shampoo

Ingredients

1 teaspoon of baking soda

¼ cup of oatmeal

1 teaspoon of lavender or other fragrant herb, crushed

Instructions

1. Combine oatmeal, baking soda and crushed lavender together in a small mixing bowl.

2. Transfer oatmeal mixture into a small grinder or a mortar and pestle.

3. Grind oatmeal mixture until thoroughly ground.

4. Transfer into a container.

5. Apply by sprinkling mixture to cover your scalp.

6. Use your hands to rub in the mixture into your scalp for 5 minutes.

7. Brush mixture out after 5 minutes.

NOTE: You can tweak ingredients ratio and produce in larger quantities.

8. Transfer remaining recipe into a container and store in a cool, dry place.

Queen's Deliciously Scented Shampoo
The fragrance of this shampoo is out of this world and only meant for Queens.

Ingredients

¼ cup liquid Castile Soap (your favorite)

¼ cup of water, distilled

10 drops of coconut fragrance oil

2 teaspoon of jojoba oil

10 drops of vanilla essential oil

Flip Cap Bottles or Foaming Bottles to dispense.

Instructions

1. Combine liquid castile soap, coconut fragrance oil, jojoba oil and water together in a mixing bowl.

2. Stir well until well combined.

3. Measure in vanilla essential oil.

4. Stir to incorporate essential oil into the mixture.

5. Transfer Shampoo mixture into a flip cap bottle.

6. Apply as you would a regular shampoo.

7. Wash hair off and pat dry.

HERBAL, ORGANIC AND ESSENTIAL OIL DIY CONDITIONER TREATMENT

Making your hair treatment right from your home has advantages that cannot be under emphasized. This hair treatment is focused on your type, texture and probably color of hair without being exposed to chemicals and additives that are synthetic, hazardous and toxic. When you condition your hair, you protect it from various hair stressors like the heat styling and harsh temperatures, poor diet, hormone irregularities and many more. When you condition your hair; a protective shield is formed over the whole hair shaft and your hair is re-moisturized, these in turn reduces the breaking of your hair.

Hair Care Blends; Choosing Carrier Oils Considering Your Kind Of Hair

Your hair has specific and peculiar needs that should be met as you make and apply every organic conditioner recipe. The information below would guide and help you to efficiently create the specific blend that will suit your hair type.

You are free to combine these oils in different ways. Make combinations of two ingredients or three or all the ingredients; whatever works for you.

a) Normal Hair Care Blends

Coconut, olive, jojoba Oils

b) Oily Hair Care Blends

Jojoba, grapeseed Oils

c) Dry/Damaged/Frizzy Hair Care Blends

Jojoba, castor, olive, coconut oils and Shea butter

d) Dandruff Fighting Hair Care Blends

Castor, avocado, sesame, olive, coconut oils

e) Thinning Hair Care Blends

Sweet almond, olive, castor, avocado, grapeseed oils

TIP: When blending oils together in the hair care blends, the percentage of avocado oil used should be 10% only; avocado oil a very difficult to wash/rinse waxy residue.

Herbal Infusion for Simple Herbal Hair Conditioner

This conditioner recipe improves the health of your hair and brightens and enhances your hair color; and should be used in place of the distilled water in the recipe below.

Blonde Hair   Dried Calendula, Chamomile, Lemon Peel

Dark Hair   Black Tea, Dried Rosemary, Cloves

Red Hair   Dried Calendula, Hibiscus, Cinnamon Bark

Gray Hair   Dried Sage, Rosemary, Thyme

Ingredients

1 tbsp each herb blend (check your type of hair above)

1/4 cup distilled water

Instructions

1. Combine three tablespoons of the herb blend that suits your hair type into a mixing bowl.

2. Measure in distilled water into the herb blend.

3. Transfer mixture to a pot.

4. Bring distilled water mixture to a boil over medium heat.

5. Take off from heat and set aside for 60 minutes, to release flavors.

6. Use a mesh strainer or cheesecloth to strain out the herbs and save the herbal infused liquid.

7. Use herbal infusion in the recipe below to substitute distilled water.

NOTE: The gray hair herbal infusion smell very "herbal", but it would give you great results over few weeks of daily usage. It is worth it all the way.

Simple Herbal Conditioner

Ingredients

½ cup of herbal infusion/distilled water

1 tsp of Carrier Oil (check table above, for your type of hair)

1 tbsp of (8g) Emulsifying Wax

Essential Oils for type of your hair

½ teaspoon of Vitamin E

5 drops of pure GSE

1 tsp of Vegetable Glycerin

Instructions

1. Combine glycerin, wax and oil together in a small bowl.

2. Stir until well combined.

3. Transfer into a glass jar, and place into a pot partly filled with water and melt over low heat.

4. Take off from heat when wax melts completely.

5. Measure in the vit. E and stir.

6. Meanwhile warm herbal infusion or distilled water in another pot or in a microwave until lukewarm.

NOTE: Step 6 is very important to the end results of your hair conditioner.

7. Pour lukewarm herbal infusion or water into the wax mixture in a slow and steady stream, using a whisk to continue stirring as you pour, until a thick, smooth and creamy consistency is reached.

8. Set mixture aside to cool.

NOTE: Mixture gets thicker as it becomes cooler.

9. Once mixture is cool, measure in pure GSE and essential oil blend.

10. Transfer mixture into 8 oz dark bottle with a good cover.

NOTE: Do not cover until mixture cools completely. As the mixture cools, shake bottle from time to time so that ingredients will not separate.

11. Keep in a dark, dry cool place.

NOTE: Decrease the carrier oil quantity and choose grapeseed oil (it happens to be light), if your hair turns out to be greasy.

Simple Hair Care Oil

This hair care oil corrects fly away ends of the hair

Ingredients

2-3 drops Jojoba oil

Instructions

1. Pour oil on your palm.

2. Put your palms against the other and rub in circles slightly.

3. Run oiled hands over your hair to straighten out fly away and frizzy hair ends.

Homemade Hair Balancing Herbal Rinse

This rinse balances the pH of your scalp, reduces the buildup of hair care products after hair conditioning. It gives your hair the shine it deserves and helps the manageability of your hair.

Importance of Herbal Rinse

1. Fights against and heals inflammation.

2. Heals chemical and synthetic hair treatments skin problems

3. Serves as a dandruff treatment.

4. Reduces hair grease.

Ingredients

Herbs (check table below)

2 cups distilled water

Dark glass container

Normal-Dry Hair: 3 tbsps dried chamomile, 3 tbsps lavender

Thinning Hair/Oily Hair/Dandruff: 3 tbsps dried peppermint, 3 tbsps rosemary

Instructions

1. Combine herb blends and distilled water together into a mixing bowl.

2. Transfer into a pot and bring to a boil over medium high heat.

3. Take off heat and set aside for 60 minutes to release flavors.

4. Use a mesh strainer or cheesecloth to strain out herbs.

5. Transfer herbal hair rinse into a dark glass bottle.

6. Apply by gently rubbing the rinse into your hair and scalp with your hands.

7. Wash out and pat dry.

Rose Jojoba Hair Conditioner

This recipe is very easy to make.

Ingredients

Makes: 1 application

1-3 drops Rosemary Essential Oil

1 tbsp Jojoba

Instructions

1. In a tiny condiment bowl, combine rosemary essential oil and jojoba essential oil together.

2. Pour into a clean and sterile glass bottle.

NOTE: The ingredients can be increased to make a larger quantity.

3. Use hair conditioner by wetting your hair with warm water and then applying the hair conditioner to your hair.

4. Let it sit in for 15 to 30 minutes before you wash off.

HERBAL, ORGANIC AND ESSENTIAL OIL DIY DEEP CONDITIONER HAIR TREATMENT

Fruity hair conditioner

Ingredients

1 Cup of coconut milk

2 tablespoon of Mango Butter/Oil

¼ Cup of Honey

Instructions

1. Combine coconut milk, mango butter and honey together into a mixing bowl.

2. Stir to combine, until well combined.

3. Transfer to a pot over medium low heat, and warm slightly.

4. Apply to slightly damp and clean hair.

5. Wrap the treated hair for 30-60 minutes with a plastic shower cap.

6. Wash off and pat hair dry.

Egg/Mayonnaise Flavored Hair Conditioner

Ingredients

2 eggs, beaten

1 cup mayonnaise

1 tbsp olive oil

Instructions

1. Combine eggs, mayonnaise and olive oil together into a small bowl.

2. Whip mixture until well mixed and a thick creamy consistency is reached.

3. Rub into your hair thoroughly to dry and clean.

4. Cover your hair with a plastic cap.

5. Use a hand-held blow drier or hood drier to dry hair for 20 minutes.

6. Wash off, pat dry and apply shampoo to your hair.

Rosewood Deep Hair Conditioner

Ingredients

5 drop sandalwood oil

5 drops lavender oil

15 drops rosewood oil

Unscented oil

Instructions

1. Combine 5 drops of sandalwood oil and 5 drops of lavender with 15 drops of rosewood oil.

2. Mix into an unscented oil.

3. Transfer mixture into a resealable plastic bag and dip into warm water to warm mixture up and wrap for about 20 minutes.

4. Apply as you would a regular shampoo

Mayonnaise/Cinnamon Hair Conditioner
This recipe hydrates your hair and gives your hair the needed shine.

Ingredients

Cinnamon

Mayonnaise

Honey

2 eggs, beaten

Few drops milk

Instructions

1. Combine cinnamon, mayonnaise, honey, eggs and a few drops of milks together into a small mixing bowl.

2. Transfer mixture to a pot and place over medium low heat until slightly warmed.

3. Apply and leave in your for 30-60 minutes.

Honeyed Mayonnaise Mix

This conditioner has so many moisturizing agents, proteins and other hair growing substances. It promotes the growth of hair and should also be used to deep-condition your lovely curls.

Ingredients

3 tablespoons Honey

4 drops of Peppermint Essential Oil

4 tablespoons of mayonnaise

EVOO

1 Egg, beaten

EVCO

4 drops of Rosemary Essential Oil

Instructions

1. Combine honey, mayonnaise, evoo, beaten egg and evco together in a small mixing bowl.

2. Mix thoroughly until well combined.

3. Measure in peppermint and rosemary essential oils.

4. Stir thoroughly until essential oils are evenly distributed in the mixture.

5. Shampoo your hair before applying mayonnaise deep conditioner treat.

6. Leave on for 60 minutes.

7. Wash off and pat dry.

Hair Glow Deep Conditioner

Ingredients

½ cup of any moisturizing conditioner as a base

1 tablespoon of honey

½ of an avocado

2 teaspoon of black Jamaican castor oil

1 tablespoon of mayonnaise

2 teaspoon of coconut oil

You can substitute the oils to fit your hairs likings!

Instructions

1. Combine moisturizing conditioner and avocado together in a small bowl.

2. Transfer into an electric blender and blend until a smooth consistency is reached.

3. Remove avocado mixture from blender.

4. Stir in honey, castor oil, mayonnaise and coconut oil into the avocado mixture.

5. Stir until well incorporated.

6. Apply to hair and leave for some minutes, covering your hair with a plastic cap.

7. Wash off and pat hair dry.

Hot Coconut Hair Mix

Use on damaged or normal hair

Ingredients

1 teaspoon of calendula oil

1 tablespoon of coconut oil

Instructions

1. Combine calendula oil and coconut oil in a small mixing bowl.

2. Transfer into a double boiler over medium low heat.

3. Heat calendula oil mixture until melted.

4. Take off heat and set aside to cool slightly.

5. Stir together and apply warm mixture to the hair.

6. Cover hair with a towel for 5 minutes.

7. Wash off with warm water and pat hair dry.

Light Cream Hair Conditioner

Ingredients

1/2 cups of coconut milk

2 tbsp of olive oil

1 to 2 cups of yogurt

2 eggs, beaten

Instructions

1. Combine oil and eggs together in a small mixing bowl.

2. Stir in coconut milk and just enough yogurts to reach desired level of conditioner's thickness.

3. Stir well until a rich creamy consistency is reached.

4. Apply hair conditioner and leave on for 30-60 minutes.

5. Cover your hair with a plastic cap.

6. Wash off and pat hair dry.

Aloe Vera Tea Conditioning Mask
This deep conditioning mask works for any hair type, gives the hair shine and softens it.

Ingredients

Aloe Vera gel

Green Tea

Coconut oil

Rosemary

Fresh ginger

Your favorite Essential oil

Instructions

1. Brew a hot cup of green tea.

2. Measure in coconut oil, rosemary, ginger and aloe vera.

3. Stir together and return to heat.

4. Bring to a boil for 5 minutes before taking off heat.

5. Set aside to cool.

6. Strain out tea bags and transfer the aloe vera liquid into a bowl.

7. Measure in the essential oil and stir to distribute evenly.

8. Apply to your hair, covering your hair ends well, leave on for 60 minutes.

9. Wash hair with warm water and pat dry.

NOTE: If coconut oil doesn't suit your hair type, feel free to substitute another oil type.

Castornnaise Deep Conditioner

This recipe is designed for a 12 inches long hair or lesser; feel free to adjust ingredients for a longer hair length

Ingredients:

1 tbsp mayonnaise

1 egg, beaten

1 tsp cold pressed castor oil

1-2 tsps olive oil

1 drop vitamin E oil

1 tbsp rinse out conditioner, if desired

Instructions

1. Combine mayonnaise, beaten egg, castor oil, olive oil and vitamin E oil together in a small mixing bowl.

2. Stir thoroughly until well combined.

3. Wash hair well before application.

4. Apply to damp hair massaging into every part of your hair and scalp.

5. Wear plastic cap.

6. Leave on for 20-30 minutes before rinsing out.

TIP: Use rinse out conditioner when rinsing out.

Honey Glow Deep Conditioner Hair Treatment

Ingredients

Some cond. (Aussie Moist)

1 1/3 cup of honey

1 cup of Coconut oil

1 inch of olive oil

3 tbsps of Lemon Juice

Instructions

1. Combine all ingredients aside the oils together into a bowl.

2. Transfer coconut and olive oil into a glass bottle.

3. Place bottle in a pot partly filled with water, and warm over medium low heat for 2 minutes.

4. Wash your hair and pour mixture on your hair before pouring the coconut/olive oil mixture also.

5. Leave on and cover your hair with a plastic cap for 30 minutes.

HERBAL, ORGANIC AND ESSENTIAL OIL DIY HAIR DETANGLER

Aloe Juice Detangler

Ingredients

6 ½ -7 ounces of Aloe Vera Juice

8 ounce Spray Bottle

3-5 drops Lemon, vanilla or sweet orange essential Oils (for fragrance), if desired

1 tablespoon of Jojoba Oil

1 tablespoon of Avocado Oil

Instructions

1. Combine aloe vera juice and the oils together in a small mixing bowl.

2. Stir together until well combined.

3. Transfer aloe juice/oil mixture into a spray bottle.

4. Add few drops of the essential oil you are using.

5. Stir mixture to evenly distribute essential oil.

6. Store in a refrigerator.

7. Shake well before each use.

Natural Aloe Vera leave in & Detangler Mix

This recipe duals as a detangler and a leave-in. Before you condition or shampoo your hair, this detangler recipe is applied.

Ingredients

3 tbsps Aloe Vera juice

1 tbsp Grapeseed oil or any of your favorite essential oil

Instructions

1. Combine aloe vera juice and grapeseed oil together in a bowl.

2. Stir well until well combined.

3. Transfer into a spray bottle.

4. Shake bottle vigorously to combine mixture well.

5. Spray your hair with a rich portion of this detangler mix, until your hair is drenched.

NOTE: Breaking your hair into different sections may be of great help.

6. Rub in detangler mix with your hands into your hair, and smoothing your hair to make certain that each hair strand is richly coated.

7. Use comb or your fingers to detangle each parted hair sections.

8. Wash hair, pat dry and style as you would regularly.

HERBAL, ORGANIC AND ESSENTIAL OIL DIY HAIR BUTTER TREATMENT

Rich Shea Hair Butter

Ingredients

Shea butter

1 tbsp olive oil,

2 tsps almond oil,

1 tsp jamacian black castor oil,

1 tsp tea tree oil,

1 tbsp coconut oil,

1 tsp vitamin e oil.

Instructions

1. Transfer shea butter into a double boiler over medium low heat.

2. Melt until completely melted.

3. Take off from heat.

4. Measure in the olive oil, coconut oiil, almond oil, castor oil, vitamin E oil and tea tree oil.

5. Stir well until thoroughly combined.

NOTE: You can use an egg beater to whisk.

Hair Butter Moisturizer

Ingredients

 Oil blend (flax seed oil, grape seed oil, olive oil, vegei oil, jojoba oil, fish oil, coconut oil,

   tea tree oil or castor oil)

   8 oz. Unrefined or Raw shea butter

Instructions

1. Combine shea butter and oils together in a large mixing bowl.

NOTE: If you are using more than 6 of the oils above; use a teaspoon each for the oil blend. If you are using less than 6 of them, you will use a tablespoon of each oil for the oil blend.

2. Transfer mixture into an electric mixer.

3. Mix until a smooth consistency is reached.

4. Transfer into a well covered container.

5. Store in a cool dry place.

Complete Hair Butter

Ingredients

10 drops of your favorite essential oil

8 ounce of unrefined organic Shea Butter

1 tablespoon of 100 percent Jojoba oil

Instructions

1. Combine jojoba oil and shea butter together in a small mixing bowl.

2. Mix with a hand mixer until well blended.

3. Measure in the essential oil.

4. Stir to distribute evenly into the mixture.

5. Transfer mixture into an airtight container

7. Apply as a sealant for your kinks and curls.

Tropical Aloe Hair Cream

Ingredients

2 heaping tbsps unrefined mango

Illipe butter

3 tbsps Tamanu oil

3 tbsps Organic Aloe Vera Juice

Shea butter

3 tbsps unrefined coconut oil

3 tbsps rosehip seed oil

8 tbsps Organic aloe Vera gel

3 tbsps olive oil

3-6 drops Vitamin E oil, unrefined

6-9 drops Tea tree oil

Instructions

1. Combine unrefined mango, illipe and shea butter together.

2. Mix well until well combined.

3. Transfer into a microwave until melted to liquid form.

4. Measure in the oils, aloe juice, aloe gel (every remaining ingredient)

5. Using a hand mixer, mix mixture until a fine creamy consistency is reached.

6. Keep in a refrigerator after application.

TIP: It can also be used as a body cream.

Hair Butter Mask with Pumpkin Seed

Ingredients

4 tablespoons pumpkin seed butter, organic

4 tablespoons extra dark Jamaican black castor oil

4 tablespoon of glycogen protein balancing conditioner

Instructions

1. Combine all ingredients together in a small mixing bowl.

2. Mix well until well combined.

3. Apply butter mask into the hair and hair strands.

4. Wear a plastic cap after application, for 60 minutes.

5. Wash off with and pat dry.

NOTE: This mask can also be used as a deep conditioner and as a detangler. If you use as a detangler, make sure you rinse out with a hair conditioner of your choice and make sure every of the mask is removed from your hair.

Cocoa Butter Hair Balm

Ingredients

1/8 cup of Saffron Oil

1 ounce or 1 stick of Cocoa Butter

3 Tablespoons of Shea Butter

1/8 - ¼ cup of Olive Oil

3 Tablespoons of Coconut oil

Instructions

1. Combine shea butter, coconut oil and cocoa butter together in a mixing bowl.

2. Mix well until very combined.

3. Transfer into a double boiler and melt over low heat until completely melted.

4. Measure in saffron and olive oil and stir.

5. Transfer into a glass jar or container, cover and refrigerate.

NOTE: This product is semi-hardened at room temperature and it dissolves easily in the palms of your hand when you want to use.

TIP: You can apply this product after using leave-in condition, and before applying any curl defining product. This moisturizes the tips of the hair and the scalp.

Hair Butter Mask

Ingredients

1 teaspoon of pure cocoa powder

2 tablespoons of melted cocoa butter

1 tablespoons of olive oil

2 tablespoons of vegetable shortening

Instructions

1. Combine cocoa powder, melted cocoa butter, olive oil and vegetable shortening together in a mixing bowl.

2. Stir well until a fine and smooth consistency is reached.

3. Apply and rub on your hair edges and hair ends.

4. Take hair out of the way by pinning it up.

5. Leave mask on for 15-30 minutes.

6. Follow with shampoo and conditioner.

HERBAL, ORGANIC AND ESSENTIAL OIL DIY HAIR OIL TREATMENT

DIY Apricot Hair oil
This hair oil work well for twists and braids

Ingredients

1oz. coconut oil

2 oz. apricot oil

1 oz. jojoba oil

1 tbsp avocado oil

1 tbsp safflower oil

Instructions

1. Combine coconut oil, apricot oil, jojoba oil, avocado and safflower oil together in a mixing bowl.

2. Stir well to combine until a smooth consistency is reached.

3. Apply by massaging a rich amount of hair oil into your hair.

DIY Olive/Coconut Hair Oil Mix

Ingredients

4 ounce of coconut oil

3 ounce of olive oil

Instructions

1. Combine coconut oil and olive oil together in a small mixing bowl.

2. Stir well to combine.

3. Transfer into a bottle with a good cover.

4. Apply four times weekly.

DIY Castor Hair Oil

Ingredients

2 oz bottle

1 oz Jamaican Black Castor Oil

Essential oil for fragrance, if desired

2 tbsps grapeseed Oil

Instructions

1. Add 1 fluid ounce of castor oil into a 2 ounce bottle.

2. Measure in grapeseed oil and the essential oils together.

3. Cover bottle and shake vigorously.

4. Apply as you would any regular hair oil.

Hot Coconut Oil Hair Mix

Ingredients

1 tablespoons of Castor Oil

2 tablespoons of Coconut Oil

1 tablespoon of Jojoba Oil

2 drops of Vitamin E Oil

1 teaspoon of Peppermint Oil

Olive oil, optional

Instructions

1. Combine all the oils together in a small bowl.

2. Stir until well combined.

3. Transfer into a double boiler and melt over low heat until completely melted.

4. Allow oils to cool slightly but not lukewarm.

5. Apply to sectioned hair, from hair ends to the root and scalp.

6. Leave on, wearing plastic cap for 10-15 minutes.

7. Condition hair.

Egg Oil Hair Mask

Ingredients

2 eggs, beaten

5 tbsps of olive oil

Instructions

1. Combine eggs and olive oil together in a small mixing bowl.

2. Mix thoroughly until well combined and a smooth creamy consistency is reached.

3. Apply by massaging into your hair.

4. Leave on and cover hair with a plastic cap for 15 minutes.

5. Wash off and pat hair dry.

Hair Growth Oil Inversion

Ingredients

2-3 tbsps coconut oil or olive oil

Instructions

1. Measure in your scalp oil of choice into a microwavable bowl.

2. Warm for few minutes until lukewarm.

3. Bending over, facing down completely for 5 minutes; massage oil into your scalp with your hands.

TIP: The bending down inversion reverses blood flowing to the scalp and results in making your hair grow.

NOTE: If you are light headed, dizzy, sick or pregnant, do not do this.

4. Apply oil inversion for 7 days.

Hair Oil Mask

Ingredients

4 tablespoons of olive oil

2 whole eggs

Instructions

1. Combine eggs and olive oil together in a small mixing bowl.

2. Mix thoroughly until well combined and a smooth creamy consistency is reached.

3. Apply by massaging into your hair.

4. Leave on and cover hair with a plastic cap for 10 minutes.

5. Wash off and pat hair dry.

Carrier Oil Herbal Hair Treat

Ingredients

1 cup organic carrier oil

3-5 tbsps of herbs of your choice

Instructions

1. Infuse oils for 2 weeks by measuring herbs into oil mixture in a jar.

2. Stir well to combine and cover well.

3. Set aside for 2 weeks until flavors have been released and the oil infused.

TIP: Shake jar vigorously on a daily basis.

4. Strain out herbs using a mesh strainer or cheesecloth.

5. Transfer herbal infused oil into a jar or container.

6. Store in a refrigerator.

NOTE: Herbal hair oil will keep for 6 months if well refrigerated.

Hair Length Oil Mix

Ingredients

3 drops cedarwood essential oil

1/8 cup jojoba oil

3 drops lemon essential oil

1/8 cup grapeseed oil

3 drops rosemary essential oil

3 drops lavender essential oil

3 drops thyme essential oil

Instructions

1. Combine jojoba oil, grapeseed oil, and all the essential oils together in a small mixing bowl.

2. Stir well to combine.

3. Apply by using your hands to massage oil mix into your scalp.

TIP: Focus hair oil mix on the affected hair loss areas.

4. Store in a dark, cool and dry place.

NOTE: Do not use rosemary essential oil if you are heavy with child.

Hot Oil Treatment for Hair Growth

Ingredients

3 drops thyme essential oil

1/8 cup jojoba oil

3 drops lavender essential oil

3 drops rosemary essential oil

1/8 cup grapeseed oil

3 drops cedarwood essential oil

Instructions

1. Combine all oils and essential oils together.

2. Stir to combine until well mixed.

3. Apply by massaging into your scalp at night.

TIP: Focus on thinning areas.

4. Wash off and pat hair dry in the morning.

Organic DIY Hot Hair Oil Treat

Ingredients

Castor Oil

Olive Oil

Instructions

1. Combine castor and olive oil together in a mixing bowl.

2. Stir well to combine.

3. Transfer into a pot and heat over medium high heat.

4. Heat until warm. Take off from heat once warm.

5. Apply to the ends of your hair to your hair root and scalp.

TIP: Organic hot hair oil treat can be used before you wash hair

6. Leave on for 60 minutes or more.

Beautiful Hair Oil

Ingredients

1 teaspoon of neem oil, if desired

1 tablespoon of castor oil

1 tablespoon of organic argan oil

Few of drops essential oils, if desired

1 tablespoon of coconut oil

1 tablespoon of olive oil

1 tablespoon of broccoli seed oil

Instructions

1. Combine neem oil, castor oil, argan oil, coconut oil, olive oil and broccoli seed oil together in a mixing bowl.

2. Stir well to combine.

TIP: You can warm the oil mixture if you like.

3. Measure in essential oils drop.

4. Stir well to incorporate.

5. Wash hair well, clean and dry well.

6. Apply to your hair and scalp by massaging with your hands.

7. Cover your hair with a plastic cap and leave mixture in hair over the night.

8. Use clarifying shampoo to wash oil mixture out of your hair and scalp; and pat dry.

TIP: Tweak ingredients to get an increase in quantity of recipe.

9. Style and condition your hair.

NOTE: Treat hair with this beautiful hair oil treat.

Hair Power Hair Oil

Ingredients

½ large bottle of Cayenne Pepper

45 cut tea bags

2-4 drops onion seed oil

30 Biotin pills, blended

1-2 drops garlic seed oil

Instructions

1. Combine cayenne pepper, tea bags and biotin pills together in a mixing bowl.

2. Stir to combine.

3. Infuse in an oven for 5 hours.

4. Take off from heat and set aside to cool to room temperature.

5. Stirring occasionally.

6. Use cheesecloth or mesh strainer to strain out the tea from the oil.

7. Measure in onion and garlic oil into the tea infused mixture.

8. Store in a dark, cool and dry place.

HERBAL, ORGANIC AND ESSENTIAL OIL DIY HAIR GROWTH TREATMENT

Mustard Hair Growth Mask

Ingredients

2 tablespoons olive oil

2 tablespoons ground mustard powder

1 egg yolk

2 teaspoons sugar

2 tablespoons hot water

Instructions

1. Combine mustard, water, egg yolk, sugar and oil together in a small mixing bowl.

2. Stir well until a smooth consistency is reached.

3. Apply to sectioned hair, massage hair growth mask into the scalp.

NOTE: Do not put to hair tips or hair ends.

4. Cover your hair with a plastic wrap or cap.

TIP: Place a hot damp towel on the plastic wrap to keep heat in. It will start burning quite fast, but its a good one. If you feel the burning might be an allergy, wash off immediately.

5. Leave on for 15-60 minutes.

6. Wash off completely with warm water and pat hair dry.

7. Apply shampoo.

NOTE: Use hair growth mask twice weekly for 4-8 weeks, for maximum results.

Essential Blend Growth Oil

Ingredients

½ teaspoon jojoba oil

3 drops lavender

2 drops rosemary

2 drops thyme

4 teaspoon grapeseed oil

Instructions

1. Combine jojoba oil, grapeseed oil and the essential oils together in an applicator/spray bottle.

2. Shake vigorously to combine.

3. Apply by massaging into the scalp for 2 minutes.

4. Cover hair with a warm damp towel.

5. Leave on for 60 minutes.

6. Wash hair out with a mild shampoo and pat dry.

TIP: Use daily for 28 weeks.

Hair Force Deep Conditioner

HFDC contains a hygroscopic substance that keeps hair moist. This recipe adds protein to your hair and in turn grows your hair and strengthens it.

Ingredients

5 drops peppermint oil

1/4 Cup olive oil

1 egg, beaten

1/8 Cup honey

1 avocado

1 teaspoon of biotin powder

Instructions

1. Combine peppermint oil, olive oil, beaten egg, honey, avocado and biotin powder together.

2. Mix to combine, until a batter-like consistency is reached.

3. Make sure hair is damp.

4. Apply a rich layer to your hair.

5. Cover your hair with a plastic cap or wrap for 30-60 minutes.

6. Wash off and pat hair dry.

Rich Herbal Infused Growth Serum

Ingredients

1 cup of distilled water

10 drops of Lavender Essential Oil

2 tbsps of Dried Nettle Leaf

10 drops of Rosemary Essential Oil

2 tbsps of Natural Aloe Vera Gel

10 drops of Clary Sage Essential Oil

2 tbsps of Horsetail Leaf (if desired)

Instructions

1. Bring distilled water to a boil.

2. Toss in horsetail and dried nettle leaf.

3. Set aside until the water becomes cool.

4. Using a mesh strainer or cheesecloth, strain out the leaves.

5. Transfer liquid into a spray bottle.

6. Measure in lavender, rosemary, clary sage essential oils and aloe vera gel into the spray bottle.

7. Shake vigorously to evenly distribute.

8. Transfer bottle into a refrigerator for 3 months.

TIP: Leave stored in the refrigerator, 3 months before usage.

9. Shake well before each use; apply by spraying richly on your hair roots, 1-2 times daily.

Hair Health Growth mixture

Ingredients

2 avacados

1-2 bananas (depends on hair length)

2 teaspoons shea butter

2 to 3 drops tea tree oil

1 drop eucalyptus oil

Instructions

1. Combine Avocado, banana and shea butter into an electric blender or food processor.

2. Blend until a smooth consistency is reached.

3. Transfer into a bowl and measure in tea tree oil and eucalyptus oil.

4. Stir well to evenly distribute.

5. Apply by using your hands to massage into your scalp and your hair.

6. Use a wide tooth comb to comb hair.

7. Leave on for 5-10 minutes.

8. Wash off and pat hair dry.

Hair Smoothie from the Caribbean

This potion leaves your hair silky, soft, smooth, strong and healthy.

Ingredients

½ avocado (ripe)

½ cup of Coconut milk

½ banana (ripe)

1 tablespoon of Castor oil

2 tablespoon of Rosemary

1 teaspoon of Cayenne Pepper

Instructions

1. Combine avocado, coconut milk, banana, castor oil, rosemary and cayenne pepper together.

2. Stir together and transfer into an electric blender.

3. Blend until a smooth consistency is reached.

4. Apply mixture to the tip of your hair, along your hair strands and down to the root and scalp.

5. Leave on for 15-60 minutes.

6. Wash off with warm water and pat hair dry.

TIP: ingredients can be tweaked, depending on the length of hair.

Apple Cider Vinegar Growth Rinse

Ingredients

2 tablespoons rosemary dried leaf

1 cup apple cider vinegar

1 cup water

Instructions

1. Measure vinegar into a small mixing bowl.

2. Add in rosemary into the mixing bowl.

3. Stir to combine and transfer into the microwave for 30 seconds.

4. Strain vinegar.

TIP: Use the smallest available strainer.

5. Add water and stir well to combine.

6. Apply as you would a regular rinse.

DIY Organic Conditioner (Hair-Growth-Stimulator)

Ingredients

¼ cup of plain natural yogurt

1 egg

1 teaspoon of fresh lemon juice

8 to 10 drops of eucalyptus oil (or olive oil, or rosemary oil, or rosemary/olive oil and canola oil)

Instructions

1. Combine yogurt, beaten egg and lemon juice together.

2. Stir to combine and transfer into an electric blender.

3. Blend until a smooth consistency is reached.

4. Apply massaging on your scalp and hair.

5. Leave on for 20-30 minutes.

6. Wash off your hair and pat dry.

DIY Coconut/Honey Cooling Hair Mask

Ingredients

Castor oil

Avocado oil

10-20 drops peppermint essential oil

Olive oil

Raw honey

Shea moisture deep conditioning mask

Organic Coconut Milk

Instructions

1. Combine castor, olive, avocado oils and honey together in a bowl.

2. Stir well until well combined.

3. Mix in the deep conditioning mask and coconut milk together into the castor/honey mixture.

4. Stir well until a smooth, thick and creamy consistency is reached.

5. Measure in peppermint essential oil.

6. Stir well to incorporate essential oil into the mixture.

7. Wash hair and pat dry.

8. Apply cooling hair mask to damp hair.

9. Leave on for 30 minutes.

10. Wash off and pat hair dry.

HERBAL, ORGANIC AND ESSENTIAL OIL DIY HAIR GEL TREATMENT

Organic Aloe Hair Gel

Ingredients

3 egg whites

1-2 tablespoons vegetable glycerin

2/3 cup aloe Vera gel

5-8 drops essential oil(s) of choice (orange and vanilla extract)

1/8 cup of water

Instructions

1. Combine egg whites, vegetable glycerin, aloe gel and water together in a small mixing bowl.

2. Transfer aloe gel mixture into an electric blender.

3. Blend for 20 seconds, until a smooth consistency is reached.

4. Transfer into a container and cover well.

5. Store in a refrigerator until you want to apply.

Aloe Pectin Hair Gel

Ingredients

1 cup aloe vera juice

1 (approx. 1.60 oz.) packet instant fruit pectin

¼ teaspoons honey

¼ teaspoons agave nectar

2 teaspoon EVOO

1 teaspoon sweet almond oil

5-7 drops of your favorite essential oils, (for fragrance), if desired

Instructions

1. Carefully and slowly add pectin in a stream into a mixing bowl.

NOTE: To avoid fruit pectin clumps, you need to make sure you are pouring slowly.

2. Stir in aloe vera juice.

3. Measure in agave nectar, honey, evoo and sweet almond oil.

4. Stir to combine until thoroughly mixed.

5. Measure in the essential oils.

6. Stir to again to evenly distribute essential oils into the aloe mixture.

7. Transfer aloe gel mixture into a bowl; cover very well.

8. Store in a refrigerator.

Chamomint Hair Styling Gel

Ingredients

   1 tablespoon lemon juice

   1/2 teaspoon xanthan gum powder

   1 tablespoon/2 teabags of chamomile

   1 cup water

   ½ tablespoon/1 teabag of mint

   1/3 cup aloe vera juice

   1 teaspoon maple syrup

Instructions

1. Bring cup of water to a boil.

2. Measure in chamomile and mint into boiling water.

3. Set aside to release tea flavors into the liquid and cool to room temperature.

4. Using a mesh strainer, tea strainer, or cheesecloth, strain out the tea from the liquid and discard teabags.

5. Measure in lemon juice, xanthan gum powder, aloe vera juice and maple syrup into the herbal tea.

6. Whisk all ingredients together.

7. Set aside to rest for a minute.

NOTE: Xanthan gum will thicken gradually.

TIP: Add a little more xanthan gum if your desired degree of thickness has not been reached, and add a little more water if it turns out too thick.

Matilda's Organic Curls Cream

Ingredients

1 jar or tube of Non-Flaking Gel or Aloe

1 tablespoon avocado oil, coconut oil, olive oil, mango butter or jojoba oil

2 tablespoons of pure shea butter,

Instructions

1. Combine aloe or non flaking gel, avocado oil, and shea butter together.

2. Mix well until a smooth consistency is reached.

3. Wash hair and apply by massaging cream into your scalp and hair with your hands.

4. Use a wide tooth brush to comb hair in, and to form definition.

5. Shake your hair and you are good.

Styling Cream Moisturizer

Ingredients

6 tbsps your favorite moisturizing conditioner

12 tbsps aloe vera gel

2 pinches cinnamon

½ tsp your favorite oil (you can use evoo)

2 tsps blue agave nectar

Tea tree or jasmine essential oils

Instructions

1. Combine your moisturizing conditioner, aloe vera gel, cinnamon, evoo oil and blue agave nectar together in a small bowl.

2. Stir thoroughly to combine until a thick consistency is reached.

TIP: The end result should be light when compared to a gel, but should have a thicker consistency than an average styling cream.

3. Transfer mixture into a glass jar.

Hair Refreshing Styling Spray

Ingredients

2 teaspoons Epsom salt

1 cup hot water

1/3 cup aloe vera gel

1 tablespoon jojoba or olive Oil

2 tablespoons Conditioner

Instructions

1. Combine epsom salt, water, aloe vera gel, jojoba oil and conditioner together.

2. Stir to combine.

3. Transfer into a spray bottle.

4. Shake vigorously before use.

5. Store in a refrigerator.

6. a) Wash hair.

   b) Apply by spraying on damp hair to style.

7. Apply by spraying on dry hair to revive and refresh the hair in the afternoon

TIP: In hot temperatures, do not use oil for this recipe; substitute with a bit of honey and/or aloe vera juice as a substitute.

NOTE: You can experiment and tweak ingredients to suit your hair type. The effectiveness of this hair styling spray depends on the brands of the products used.

Glowing Waves Coconut Milk/Oil Conditioner

This recipe is a conditioner that helps to moisturize your curls. Works well for all hair type, gives your hair, strength; and gives an out of this world kinda glow. It remedies hair loss and stimulates hair growth.

Ingredients

1 tablespoon your favorite hair conditioner

1 tablespoon cane molasses

3 tablespoon coconut milk (or add to taste)

1 tablespoon coconut oil

1 tablespoon honey

1 tablespoon rosemary infused olive oil

Instructions

1. In a small bowl, combine your favorite hair conditioner, cane molasses, coconut milk, coconut oil, honey and rosemary infused olive oil together.

2. Stir to combine, until thoroughly combined.

3. Shampoo hair 3 days before applying hair mixture.

4. Apply mixture by massaging from your hair tips to the roots and scalp.

5. Leave on for 60 minutes or more.

NOTE: You can substitute the olive oil for any other oil of your choice.

DIY Leave-In Conditioner

This recipe fights against hair loss, dandruff, dry and itchy scalp, and it promotes hair growth.

Ingredients

10 small squirts of Lime Juice

½ cup of Aloe Juice and gel

1 cup distilled water

Milk/Water from 1 coconut

1 tablespoon of melted Shea butter

1 tablespoon of melted Coconut Oil

1 teaspoon of Olive oil

½ teaspoon of Thyme oil

1 teaspoon of Rosemary oil

Instructions

1. Combine lime juice, aloe gel & juice, distilled water, coconut milk, melted shea butter, melted coconut oil, olive oil, thyme oil and rosemary oil together in a small bowl.

2. Mix until a smooth consistency is reached.

3. Transfer leave -in conditioner into a spray bottle.

4. Apply as you would a regular leave-in conditioner.

Protein Filled Mud mask

This recipe grows and strengthens your hair, brings hair back into form and gives time trusted elasticity

Ingredients

1 cup aloe vera juice/coconut milk

2 cups Nupur henna mixture (see below)

Your favorite moisture rinse out conditioner

1 large egg, beaten

2 1/2 tbsps coconut oil

4 tbsps agave nectar/honey

Instructions

1. Combine ayurvedic henna mixture with coconut milk or aloe vera juice together in a bowl.

2. Stir well until well combined.

3. Measure in the coconut oil, beaten egg and the moisture rinse out conditioner.

4. Stir well to evenly distribute.

5. Apply by massaging into your hair ends, hair strands, hair roots and scalp.

6. Leave on for 60-180 minutes.

7. Cover hair with a plastic cap or wrap

8. Wash off with water and a protein-free, rich in moisture conditioner.

TIP: This gives your hair a glowing and popping feel.

NOTE: a) Avoid bending, much movement that may affect the position of your hair while the mud mask is still in your hair. This prevents hair from knotting and tangling. b) Ayurvedic henna mixture (Brahmi, hibiscus powder, shikakai, aloe vera, amla, bhringraj, neem, and jatamansi powders).

HERBAL, ORGANIC AND ESSENTIAL OIL DIY NATURAL SHAVING CREAM

Homemade Shaving Cream

This shaving cream makes your skin luxuriantly pampered with this recipe. It's a great alternative for those with skins that are sensitive.

Ingredients

4 tablespoons solid shea butter

3 tablespoons coconut oil

2 tablespoons sweet almond oil

10-12 drops pure lavender essential oil, if desired

Instructions

1. Mix coconut oil and shea butter together

2. Transfer into a double boiler over very low heat and melt.

3. Stir from time to time. Take mixture off heat once mixture has melts totally.

4. Measure in lavender oil and almond and stir to incorporate oils well.

5. Pour mixture into a bowl and refrigerate to allow mixture solidify.

6. Whip shaving cream mixture using an electric mixer or a stand mixer.

7. Set whipped mixture aside before you transfer in a well covered jar or container.

TIP: Do not use beyond a month.

DIY Shaving Cream

Ingredients

Makes: 2 cups

   1/2 (4 ounce) cup of coconut oil

   1/4 cup olive oil

   1/2 (4 ounce) cup shea butter

   20-25 drops eucalyptus essential oil

Instructions

1. Combine shea butter and coconut oil in a mixing bowl.

2. Transfer bowl mixture into a double boiler over medium low heat and melt.

3. Once melted, take off from heat and transfer to a bowl.

4. Measure olive oil into the mixture and stir to incorporate.

5. Refrigerate until mixture solidifies.

6. Remove from the refrigerator.

7. Using a hand mixer or standing mixer, whip bowl's mixture until stiff peaks are formed, for 3 minutes.

8. Meanwhile, as you whip mixture, measure in the essential oils.

9. Transfer whipped shaving cream into a well covered jar and store.

HERBAL, ORGANIC AND ESSENTIAL OIL DIY COCONUT OIL RECIPES FOR HAIR TREATMENT

The ultimate shine product, coconut oil! This organic all-in-one hair care product is loaded with lauric acid, anti-microbial properties, and medium chain fatty acids that gives hair strength, grows your hair and conditions your scalp. Coconut oil is loaded with minerals, vitamins and many other nourishments, nutrients and benefits for your hair.

Coconut Oil Hair Conditioner

Ingredient

1/4 tsp coconut oil, warmed (for thinner, shorter hair), 1/2 tsp coconut oil (for thicker, longer hair)

Instructions

1. Warm coconut oil.

2. Transfer into the palm of your hands.

3. Apply to hair shaft and hair ends, smoothing with your hands.

TIP: For a damaged or dry hair, measure 3-4 drops of geranium and/or sandalwood essential oils.

They serve as a leave-in and deep conditioners.

Coconut Oil Scalp Conditioner and Hair Growth Serum

Ingredients

1 tsp coconut oil

Instructions

1. Apply by massaging on the scalp using your hands as you massage, pressing gently.

2. Continue massage for 10 minutes.

TIP: Apply 3-4 times weekly.

Coconut Oil Anti-Dandruff

Ingredients

5 drops lavender, thyme, wintergreen or tea tree essential oils

2 tsps coconut oil

Instructions

1. Combine coconut oil and one of the essential oils above into a small bowl.

2. Stir until well blended.

3. Apply by massaging well into your scalp; cover your whole scalp-hair area.

4. Leave on, covering with a plastic cap and stay in the sun for 20-30 minutes.

TIP: This increases heat, or use a hand dryer.

Coconut Oil Frizz Tame

Ingredients

1/4-1 tsp coconut oil (depends on hair length)

Instructions

1. Warm oil.

2. Pour into the palm of your hands.

3. Apply by smoothing oil from hair ends to hair roots.

4. Use a hand dryer to blow dry your hair.

TIP: Can be used as a detangler, note, and use a little if you have short and thin hair. You can also leave the oil on to act as a sunscreen for your hair.

Coconut Oil Lice Prevention & Cure Leave-In Conditioner

Ingredients

3 tbsps coconut oil

1 tsp ylang ylang oil

1 tsp tea tree oil

1 tsp anise oil

1 cup distilled water

2 cups apple cider vinegar

Instructions

TIP: Double recipe for a fuller, longer hair (hair passing the shoulder).

1. Combine first four ingredients together in a small mixing bowl.

2. Apply by massaging oils over the entire scalp and hair area on your head.

3. Work through your hair with a comb or your fingers.

4. Leave on for 120 minutes.

5. Cover hair with a plastic cap.

TIP: Use hair dryer or stay under the sun for heat.

6. After waiting time, comb hair.

7. Wash hair well and pat dry.

8. Combine water and vinegar into a spray bottle.

9. Shake vigorously to mix.

10. Apply to hair as you rub in gently into your hair

11 Rinse hair one more time and comb.

12. Apply light coconut oil to hair, cover with a plastic cap and style your hair.

TIP: Leave on till you wash your hair again.

Coconut Oil Hair Shampoo

Ingredients

1 cup liquid castile soap

1/3 cup coconut oil

1/3 cup coconut milk

50-60 drops essential oils (lavender, peppermint, wild orange, lemon grass, clary sage and rosemary)

Instructions

1. Combine coconut milk and coconut oil together.

2. Stir well until combined.

3. Warm over very super low heat.

NOTE: If heat is too high, nutrients in the mixture would be destroyed.

4. Transfer into a container.

5. Measure in castile soap and shake bottle vigorously.

6. Measure in the essential oil(s).

7. Shake bottle to incorporate.

8. Cover well.

9. Apply by squeezing on hair as you wash hair and rinse out well.

Coconut Oil Hair Conditioner

Ingredients

2/3 cup coconut oil

1 tbsp Jojoba oil

1 tbsp vitamin E oil

10 drops of your favorite essential oil

Instructions

1. Combine coconut oil, jojoba oil, vitamin E oil and any of your favorite essential oil in a mixing bowl.

2. Mix well to combine, using a hand mixer until a creamy and smooth consistency is reached.

3. After shampooing, apply 1-2 tsps of the coconut oil conditioner to hair and smooth through your hair.

4. Wash off and pay hair dry

NOTE: If you use hair dyes, coconut oil will fade the hair dye, especially red hair tint. Other hair tints/dyes may not fade.

Coconut Oil Dark Hair Color Base
For darker hair color

Ingredients

2 tbsps coconut oil

1 tbsp spent grounds

1 cup strong coffee

Instructions

1. Combine all ingredients together in a small mixing bowl

2. Stir to combine well.

3. Apply by massaging into hair.

4. Leave on for 45-60 minutes.

5. Wash off, pat dry and style your hair as desired.

Coconut Oil Blonde Hair Color Base

Ingredients

1/2 cup strong chamomile tea

1/4 cup fresh lemon juice

1/4 cup coconut oil

Instructions

1. Combine all ingredients together in a small bowl.

2. Stir to combine and transfer into an electric blender.

3. Blend until mixture emulsifies.

4. Apply to you entire hair length, tip and roots.

5. Wear plastic cap and leave on for 45-75minutes.

TIP: For added heat, stay in the sun or use hair dryer for the duration of leave-on time.

HERBAL, ORGANIC AND ESSENTIAL OIL DIY HAIR CARE RECIPES

For Oily Hair

Ingredients

10 drops lime oil, ylang ylang, and rosemary oils

¼ cup (2 oz.) unscented oil

Instructions

1. Combine 10 drops of lime oil, ylang ylang oil and rosemary oil.

2. Combine with 2 oz. of unscented oil (about 1/4 cup).

3. Apply to scalp 2 to 3 times in a week.

4. Wash out after a while.

Scented Hair Aromatherapy Recipe

This recipe gives a lovely fragrance to your hair.

Ingredient

1 drop of Lavender/Rosemary/Sandalwood

Instructions

1. Choose any one of the essential oils listed in the ingredient list.

2. Apply 1 drop to the bristles of a hair brush.

3. Use hair brush to brush your hair thoroughly.

Dandruff Scalp Treatment

This recipe combats fungi and absorbs excessive moisture on the skin.

Ingredients

1-2 tsps salt

Few drops of water

Instructions

1. Apply by sprinkling salt on your scalp.

2. Moisten your hands with water and massage scalp thoroughly with wet hands for 10-15 minutes.

3. Wash, pat dry your hair. Apply hair conditioning cream.

Anti-Dandruff Hair Oil

Ingredients

5 drops rosemary oil

5 drops lavender oil

3 tbsps unscented oil

Instructions

1. Combine 5 drops of rosemary oil and 5 drops of lavender oil together.

2. Mix with 3 tbsps of unscented oil.

3. Apply by massaging into your scalp.

4. Shampoo it out after 10 minutes.

END

Thank you for reading my book.

Thanks!

Cadhla Marielle Davids